# THE

# MEDITERRANEAN

# DIET MEAL PREP

*130 Healthy Recipes for Lasting Weight Loss and
4 Week Meal Plan*

**By**

**Julia Marino**

# TABLE OF CONTENTS

INTRODUCTION................................................................................................1

CHAPTER 1 THE MEDITERRANEAN DIET.............................................3

CHAPTER 2 HEALTH BENEFITS OF THE MEDITERRANEAN DIET...............4

CHAPTER 3 FOODS TO EAT AND AVOID.................................................6

CHAPTER 4 PLANNING THE MEDITERRANEAN DIET.......................10

CHAPTER 5 SHOPPING FOR THE MEDITERRANEAN DIET............13

CHAPTER 6 LOSE MORE WEIGHT AND LIVE HEALTHY WITH THE MEDITERRANEAN DIET..............................................................................15

CHAPTER 7 4 WEEK MEAL PLAN...........................................................19

CHAPTER 8 BREAKFAST AND STARTERS RECIPES..........................74

CHAPTER 9 APPETIZERS RECIPES.........................................................91

CHAPTER 10 MAIN AND SECOND COURSES RECIPES...................107

CHAPTER 11 SNACKS RECIPES.............................................................153

CHAPTER 12 DESSERT RECIPES...........................................................167

CONCLUSION.............................................................................................201

# INTRODUCTION

The Mediterranean diet is a lifestyle— one where you slow down and eat lots of fresh food. Very specifically, the diet is a modern set of guidelines influenced by southern Italy's traditional eating patterns, the Greek island of Crete and other areas of Greece. This way of life was first studied in the 1960s, and in 2010, the United Nations Educational, Scientific and Cultural Organization (UNESCO) properly recognized that diet pattern as part of Italy, Greece, Spain, and Morocco's cultural heritage. A more rural culture among all these regions is a common thread.

The Mediterranean Sea has long played a major role in the civilizations that it is surrounded by. It is linked by the narrow (14 mile wide) Strait of Gibraltar in the west to the Atlantic Ocean and by the Dardanelles and the Bosporus in the east to the Sea of Marmara and the Black Sea. Encircled by the coastlines of 21 countries — Algeria, Croatia, Cyprus, Egypt, France, Greece, Italy, Libya, Malta, Montenegro and Spain, to name but a few— it was a significant path for merchants and travelers, and a primary originator of food for the civilizations that have sprung up around it. The Mediterranean climate, hot and dry in the summers and cool and rainy in the winter, lends itself to crops such as olives, figs, and grapes; and the rugged, coastal landscape is more appropriate for cattle, goats, and chicken than the staple of traditional western diets: beef. The local sea offers plenty and variety of seafood.

The Western world has long been fascinated and inspired by this region in terms of governance, philosophy, science, mathematics, art, architecture and more. Currently, studies that draw direct links between what is called the Mediterranean diet and reduced heart disease complications, reduced cancer incidence and cancer deaths, and reduced incidence of Parkinson's and Alzheimer's diseases have given people another reason to support the diet.

The Mediterranean diet is based on fruits and vegetables, lean sources of protein, and healthy fats— hallmarks of most healthy diets.

The Mediterranean Diet Cookbook helps in making it easy to switch to a Mediterranean diet with quite a number of recipes that are easy to follow, tasty and delicious. These recipes are healthy and involve fresh whole food that are low in fat, carbohydrates, and have high disease-fighting nutrients and antioxidants. The Mediterranean Diet Meal Prep contains the latest research and clear instructions on how to create your personal diet meal plan, potential health benefits of the diet, as well as myth busting on what foods to eat and which ones to avoid. The Mediterranean Diet Meal Prep embraces good health and healthy eating, consisting of delicious and healthy recipes that will contribute in weight loss, hormonal balance and helps you in reinventing your life for a new and improved **YOU**.

# CHAPTER 1
# THE MEDITERRANEAN DIET

The Mediterranean diet consists of whole, non-processed foods which are rich in a large variety of vitamins and nutrients that are health promoting. This diet is the ideal plan for weight control and longtime heart health. It contains foods eaten in Spain, Southern Italy, Greece and other countries that surround the Mediterranean Sea. The emphasis lays on eating foods like beans, fish, vegetables, fruits, whole grain and high fiber breads, olive oil and nuts. Cheese, meat and sweets are limited. The foods recommended are foods which are rich in fiber, monounsaturated fats, omega-3 fatty acids.

Like any other heart-healthy diets, this recommends eating plenty of vegetables, fruits and high fiber grains. The only exception in the Mediterranean diet is that an average of 35% to 40% of calories can come from fats. Most other heart-healthy diet guidelines recommend getting less than 35% of calories from fats. The fats approved are mostly from unsaturated oils like olive oil, fish oil and certain seed oils (such as flax seed oil, soybean or canola) and nut oils (such as walnuts, almonds and hazelnuts). These oils may have a protective effect on the heart.

The Mediterranean diet is a well-balanced diet which includes complex carbohydrates and healthy fats. It offers the best solution to lose weight without sacrificing your health. Pairing it with lowered stress and increased exercise, you would not only lose weight, but you would also reduce your blood sugar, cholesterol and blood pressure.

# CHAPTER 2
# HEALTH BENEFITS OF THE MEDITERRA-NEAN DIET

For many years now, researchers have studied plenty of diets and meal philosophies for distinct health advantages and benefits for human beings which you can find summarized here below.

### A. THE MEDITERRANEAN DIET KEEPS YOU AGILE

As an older adult, the nutrients gained in a Mediterranean diet reduce your risk of having weak muscles and other frailty by an estimated 70 percent.

### B. IT REDUCES THE RISK OF PARKINSON'S DISEASE AND ALZHEIMER'S DISEASE

Research suggests that the Mediterranean diet helps improve blood sugar levels, cholesterol and general blood vessel health, which in turn helps reduce your risk of dementia or Alzheimer's disease. The high levels of antioxidants in the Mediterranean diet helps in preventing your cells from going through a damaging process of oxidative stress- this can reduce the risk of Parkinson's disease by half.

### C. IT HELPS PREVENT STROKES AND HEART DISEASE

When you follow a Mediterranean diet, it limits your intake of processed foods, red meat, refined breads and it supports drinking of red wine instead of hard liquor or rum. All these factors help prevent stroke and heart diseases.

## D. IT HELPS PROTECT AGAINST TYPE 2 DIABETES

The Mediterranean diet is rich in fiber which takes time to digest, helping to maintain a healthy weight and preventing blood sugar spikes or dips.

## E. IT HELPS INCREASE LONGETIVITY

A Mediterranean diet helps by lowering your risk of developing a heart disease or cancer and reduces your chances of death at any age by 20 percent.

## F. IT HELPS IN WEIGHT LOSS AND MAINTENANCE

A Mediterranean diet focuses on whole, fresh foods and may help you lose weight in a sustainable way.

## G. PEOPLE WITH RHEUMATOID ARTHRITIS MAY BENEFIT FROM THE MEDITERRANEAN DIET

The Rheumatoid Arthritis (RA) is an autoimmune disease whereby the immune system of the body accidentally attacks the joints which, as a result, creates pain and swelling around and in the joints. Some properties of the Mediterranean diet which includes its richness in anti-inflammatory omega-3 fatty acids help relieve symptoms of Rheumatoid Arthritis.

## H. THE MEDITERRANEAN DIET IS PROTECTIVE AGAINST SOME TYPES OF CANCER

Research suggests that the Mediterranean diet helps reduces certain types of cancer such as colorectal cancer, breast cancer and helps prevent cancer-related death. These observed beneficial effects are mainly driven by higher intakes of vegetables, whole grains and fruits.

# CHAPTER 3
# FOODS TO EAT AND AVOID

Plant-based foods like vegetables, fruits, legumes, whole grains, nuts, seeds and healthy fats like olive oil should be worked into every meal whenever possible. Below is a break-down of six exceptional components of the Mediterranean diet.

## 1. VEGETABLES

These are plant-based foods which are nutritious, colorful, healthy and extremely versatile. They can be eaten raw, grilled, boiled, pickled, sautéed, steamed and roasted. In any of these forms, vegetables should be included in your every meal. They can easily be mixed into eggs, spread over pizza or made as salad.

## 2. HEALTHY GRAINS

Healthy grains can be taken as breakfast, lunch or dinner. Whole grains are full of fiber, anti-inflammatory properties and antioxidants. A 2015 research in JAMA internal medicine linked whole grains to a lower mortality rate, most especially from chronic disease like type-2 diabetes and cardiovascular disease. Common, modern types of whole grain include oats and brown rice. While we have the ancient grains like quinoa, faro, amaranth, buckwheat, and bulgur which pack the added benefit of being gluten-free.

## 3. FRUITS

Healthy fruits included in the Mediterranean diet are avocados, grapes, olives, and figs- all these consist of antioxidants and fiber.

Try to eat as many types of fruits as possible from local sources and when seasonal. If you are considering when in the day to eat fruits, focus on when you normally would crave for a sugar fix like in the afternoon or after dinner.

## 4. PROTEINS

Good proteins to consume include shellfish and fish, especially varieties of fish which contains omega-3 fatty acids. Some of the healthiest sea foods you can consume are arctic char, mackerel, salmon, oysters and anchovies. Not forgetting plant-based proteins such as seeds, nuts, legumes and beans. These foods consist of fiber, unsaturated fats, and add instant texture and flavor to salad and can as well stand alone as satisfying snacks.

## 5. HEALTHY FATS

The elementary healthy fat of the Mediterranean diet is olive oil and it is used for cooking, sauces, vinaigrettes, baking and lots more. Supplementary to olive oil, the American Heart Association recommends healthy cooking oils like peanut, safflower and canola.

## 6. RED WINE

Health benefits of red wine are particularly noteworthy. A 2015 study published in the Annals of Internal medicine connected one serving of red wine daily (150ml. or 5 oz.) to a good increase of cholesterol in the body. Sipping a glass of wine can help to destress you while it also enhances the flavor of your food.

## UNHEALTHY FOODS TO AVOID

On the other hand, you should try to avoid at best the following two unhealthy things.

## 1. RED MEAT

You should personally have a beef with red meat. People generally consume too much red meat. For example, we have bacon or sausage for breakfast, a hot dog or hamburger for lunch, and probably steak for dinner and then wake up and do it all again. This is not healthy at all. Too much consumption of red meat has been linked to the following:

- ❖ Heart disease
- ❖ Chronic inflammation
- ❖ Dehydration
- ❖ Diabetes
- ❖ Elevated cholesterol

In addition, red meat may also contain:

- ❖ PCBs (they are toxic)
- ❖ Protein prions (which have been linked to bovine spongiform encephalopathy which is also known as mad cow disease)
- ❖ Bacteria
- ❖ Hormones
- ❖ Viruses
- ❖ Heterocyclic amines (these have been linked to cancer)

## 2. MILK

One of the most prevalent American myths is the health benefit of drinking at least three or more glasses of milk daily. Due to its saturated fat, it has a high increase in cholesterol. Whole milk has been a good and active contributor to the obesity epidemic in America and other developed nations worldwide. Three 8 oz. glasses of milk a day gives 450 calories and 15 grams of saturated fat. The hormones cows are given to increase their milk production and also the antibiotics cows are fed to prevent infection, have been found in the bloods of milk drinkers.

Regular consumption of milk may increase the risk of:

- ❖ Multiple sclerosis
- ❖ Prostate cancer
- ❖ Ovarian cancer
- ❖ Diabetes
- ❖ Heart disease
- ❖ GI disturbances due to lactose intolerance

If at all you must consume milk, taking almond milk or fat-free milk in moderation makes more sense. Likewise, take fat-free or low-fat cheese, choose fat-free or low-fat yogurt, also switch from taking butter and margarine to olive oil or a trans-free vegetable spread for your other daily dairy needs. Lastly for the ice cream junkies out there, consider taking fresh fruit sorbet or fat-free ice milk- your heart will thank you!

However, don't lose your *whey*. Dairy isn't all bad. Whey, which was once referred as a waste by product of cheese manufacturing, it is now prized as a high-quality, protein-packed snack which is low in fat and it is easily digestible.

Regular dairy products contain lactose, which is milk sugar, but whey is actually lactose free and a very good choice for people who are lactose intolerant. A whey protein smoothie or shake can be used as a substitute meal or as a snack several times in a week.

Other foods to avoid:

- ❖ Added sugar like candies, soda, table sugar, ice cream and lots more.
- ❖ Refined oils such as canola oil, cottonseed oil, soybean oil etc.
- ❖ Highly processed foods
- ❖ Refined grains like pasta made with refined wheat, white bread etc.
- ❖ You have to read food labels carefully if you want to avoid taking any of these unhealthy ingredients.

# CHAPTER 4
# PLANNING THE MEDITERRANEAN DIET

The good thing about the Mediterranean diet is that is a style of eating that is against a set of rigid rules. This means that you can customize the plan to suit your personal preferences. There is no following of a particular set of rules or going off board and feeling like a failure or loser. Notwithstanding, here are some basic tips to guide you.

## EAT MORE FISH AND LESS RED MEAT

The go-to protein in a Mediterranean diet is fish. This diet mainly emphasizes on fatty fish such as sardines, salmon and mackerel because they are very rich in brain and heart-healthy omega-3 fatty acids. Even fish that have less fat and are leaner like cod or tilapia are worth it because it still provides a good source of protein. If you currently don't get a lot of fish in your diet, an easy entry point is to assign one day in each week as fish night. Cooking fish in foil packets or parchment paper is no big deal at all and it is a no-mess way to put dinner on the table. As an alternative, you can try incorporating it in some of your favorite foods like soups, tacos and stir-fries.

## SNACK ON NUTS

Nuts are also type of Mediterranean staples. Having with you a handful of nuts whether it is cashew nut, pistachios, almond nuts or groundnuts can make a satisfying on the go snack. A study in a nutritional journal shows that if people actually substitute their standard regular snack (cookies, chips, chocolates, cereal bars, crackers, snack mix) with nuts, their diets would be lower in empty calories, added sugar and sodium. In addition, nuts consist of more minerals (such as potassium) and fiber, than processed snack foods.

## COOK WITH OLIVE OIL

Use more virgin olive oil as the oil you cook with because it is rich in heart-healthy polyunsaturated and monounsaturated fat, so you can feel good and relaxed about keeping a bottle handy in your kitchen. It can also be used in cold applications for making of salad dressing or to drizzle on side dishes or cooked vegetables.

## EAT VEGETABLES ALL DAY LONG

If you take a look at your diet and notice there is hardly any green to it, this is a good opportunity to fill it with more veggies. A nice way to do this is to eat a serving at snack time, like making a handful of spinach in a smoothie, or crunching on bell pepper strips and also a serving at dinner time. Target at least two servings of vegetables in a day. More is better- at least three servings can help to reduce stress.

## HELP YOURSELF TO WHOLE GRAINS

Help yourself to "real" grains that are still in their "whole" form and haven't gone through the refinery process. Quinoa makes a great side dish for weeknight meals and it cooks up in just 20 minutes. Barley is rich in fiber, filling, and it can be paired with mushrooms for a steamy and satisfying soup. A steaming hot bowl of oatmeal is perfect for breakfast on a cold winter morning. As surprising as it may seem, even popcorn is whole grain-you just have to keep it healthy by forgoing the butter and eating air-popped corn. You can supplement your intake with other whole grain products like whole grain pasta and bread. When grocery shopping, look out for products with the term "whole" or "whole grain" written on the food package and in the list of ingredient and if you still find it too hard to make a switch from your whole refined favorites, you can start by using whole grain blends of rice or pastas or by mixing half of a whole grain and half of a refined one.

## SIP A LITTLE WINE

The people living along the Mediterranean like the French, the Italian, the Greek, the Spanish, are ones to embrace wine but it doesn't mean you should pour it at your own leisure. Experts and dieticians who developed the Mediterranean diet for the New England journal of Medicine study advised that men should stick to a 5 oz. serving, and women to a 3 oz. serving per day. When you do sip, try to do that with a meal and it is even better if that meal is shared with your loved ones. If it happens that you are a teetotaler, you should not start to drink just for the sake of this diet.

## ENJOY EATING FRUITS FOR DESSERT

Fresh fruit is a flourishing way to satisfy your sweet tooth and it is generally a good source of fiber, antioxidants and Vitamin C. If fruits help you to eat more, add a little sugar-drizzle slices of pear with honey or you can sprinkle a little quantity of brown sugar on grapefruit. Keep fresh fruit in a visible place at home and keep a few pieces at work so you can have a healthy snack for when your stomach starts growling. Most grocery stores stock exotic fruits, so try to endeavor to pick a new one to try each week and expand your fruity horizon.

## SAVOR EVERY BITE

Eating a Mediterranean diet is as much a lifestyle as it is a diet. Instead of just gobbling down your meal all alone in front of a TV, just slow down and sit down and enjoy your meal and you can as well invite your family to savor your meal with you. Not only will you appreciate your meal and some company, eating slowly allows you to tune in to your body's fullness and hunger signals. You become more apt to eat just until you're satisfied rather than until you're busting at the seams full.

# CHAPTER 5
# SHOPPING FOR THE MEDITERRANEAN DIET

Y ou have the knowledge of the Mediterranean diet already and now it is time to put what you've learnt into practice. Firstly, start by stocking up your pantry with the best Mediterranean diet foods, starting from the healthiest seeds and nuts to the healthiest seafood. When next you visit the farmers' market or grocery store, refer to this handy shopping list.

**Vegetable Ideas:** eggplant, fennel, peppers, kale, cucumbers, sweet potatoes, artichokes, onions, leeks, garlic, radishes, shallots, Swiss chard, arugula, beets.

**Fruit Ideas:** oranges, apricots, grapes, pears, cherry, pomegranate, avocado, figs, tomatoes, olives, dates.

**Whole Grain Ideas:** barley, faro, wheat berries, quinoa, bulgur.

**Fat Ideas:** safflower, extra virgin olive oil, canola oil.

**Dairy Ideas:** Greek yoghurt, goat cheese, ricotta, Haloumi, feta, Parmigiano-Reggiano.

**Protein Ideas:** fresh mackerel or salmon, oysters, mussels. Canned anchovies, tuna, salmon. Lean game meats like bison, duck and quail.

**Legumes:** examples are peanuts, split beans, chickpeas, cannellini beans, fava beans, lentils.

**Nut and Seed Ideas:** pine nuts, walnuts, sesame seeds, almonds.

**Condiments and Spices Idea:** turmeric, hummus, fig spread, ground coriander, Spanish paprika (also known as pimento), tahini, harissa, tapenade, pesto, Zaatar, ground cumin, saffron threads.

# CHAPTER 6
# LOSE MORE WEIGHT AND LIVE HEALTHY WITH THE MEDITERRANEAN DIET

The Mediterranean diet helps you to lose weight. While some people have the fear that following a diet like this, which is relatively rich in fats like olive oil, avocados and some cheese, will make them fat, but research upon research suggests that the opposite is true. Of course, the aspect you chose and how it compares to your current diet has a role to play in that. For example, if you build a 'calorie deficit' into your meal plan, eating fewer calories than your daily recommended maximum or shedding off some fats by exercising, you should lose a few pounds. You have to burn more calories than you consume. How quickly you lose them or whether you lose some fats at all is totally up to you. If you want to lose weight and follow a Mediterranean diet, below are few tips that work.

**Eat vegetables cooked in olive oil as a main course**

When you eat a vegetable dish which is cooked in olive oil and tomato, not only is it satisfying, but you are also taking in 3-4 servings of vegetables in just one sitting. These dishes are low in carbs and they consist of low-calorie level. Accompany this meal with a piece of feta cheese and you are good to go. Another extra advantage of eating vegetable as a main course meal is that since it is not a meal enriched with carbs, you will enjoy the sleep that follows.

## Eat your main meal early in the day

Generally, in a Mediterranean diet, the main meal is lunch and it is consumed between 1pm to 3pm. By eating a larger meal early in the day, the risk of over-eating later in the day is reduced. As a matter of fact, a Spanish study showed that the number of people who ate their largest meal before 3pm lost more weight. Most people eat large meals and snack in the evening and this habit or lifestyle is one of the causes as to why obesity is a major public health threat.

## Consume the right amount of olive oil

Increasing amounts research confirm what we in the Mediterranean already know, which is that good fat doesn't make someone fat. The calories count, but in order to maintain a vegetable-based diet, you need to add to it something to provide flavor and satiety, of which is olive oil. Olive oil doesn't only make the vegetables delicious, it also helps in making the meal filling. However, this doesn't mean you should be mindlessly pouring olive oil on every single thing. A good amount which still contains all the health benefits is 3 tablespoons a day.

## Drink water mostly and sometimes coffee, tea and wine

Though it is standard in some countries like the United States to take meals with milk, is it really necessary? No, it isn't. Following the Mediterranean diet most dairy comes from yoghurt and cheese, so save your calories and put them to use by eating more of solid foods rather than eating liquid foods. The same thing applies to juice, you really don't need juice. The vitamins provided in juice can as well be gotten from fruits, which are rich in fiber and nutrients, and are also very filling. Coffee and wine each have their own place in the Mediterranean diet, but they do not replace water. Wine has been associated with various health benefits and so has been traditional Greek coffee.

## Exercise

Exercise is a required part of the Mediterranean diet, but it really doesn't have to feel like exercise, meaning it doesn't have to be strenuous. Walking often is a central aspect of the Mediterranean diet and it is a good place to start your exercise. General movement of your body throughout the day is important- it is not just enough to spend an hour every morning in the gym then afterwards just sit in your office or on the couch for the rest of the day. Implement walking breaks, do some stretches every now and then, do some house chores and if you can walk somewhere, do so instead of driving. We should try to exercise more often as exercise lowers blood pressure in a couple of ways. One way is that exercise supports weight loss specifically by reduction fat across the body, including abdominal fat. The fat in this area is associated with elevated level of a protein named angiotensinogen, and this can lead to hypertension. Exercise also assists in strengthening the heart and it makes the cardiovascular system work more efficiently by relaxing and dilating blood vessels. If you exercise to ease yourself of stress rather than raiding the refrigerator, you will not only eliminate emotional eating, but you would also maintain a healthy weight.

## Eat smart

We must learn to eat smart and this can be done initially by monitoring the portions of food we consume. As the years pass by, packaged food portions and restaurant food portions have been increased in size. The weight of an average bagel now is about four to five oz., which is equal to four or five slices of bread. Cookies now weigh about the same size as a saucer. And a portion of pasta in a restaurant would have, in the past, fed a family of four. To estimate what an average serving of a packaged food is, look out for the nutritional label information. You'll probably be surprised to find out that the 'single' food package you thought was for just one person is actually meant for two or more people. You necessarily don't need to measure and weigh food, but you can use your common sense or intuition and learn to use your eyeball to correct portions. Take for example, a piece of meat weighing three oz. is about the size and thickness of a deck of cards and a medium-sized orange is just about the same size as a tennis ball. It is the standard of food, not the amount that makes a good meal.

Additionally, we can also eat smart by eating less processed foods like trans fats, refined sugar and saturated fats, and replacing these processed foods with healthier foods that have lower calories and high fiber contents like fruits, vegetables, olive oil, monounsaturated fats, omega-3 fats etc. Trans-fats are associated with rapid weight gain, and so should be avoided.

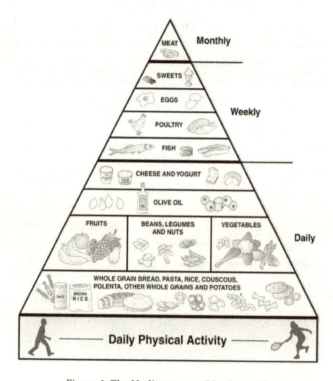

Figure 1: The Mediterranean Diet Pyramid

# CHAPTER 7
# 4 WEEK MEAL PLAN

E njoy the delicious flavors of eating Mediterranean and losing weight with this healthy meal plan. This is a full 28-day plan of delicious, healthy, nutritious Mediterranean inspired snack and meals which make it easy to stay right on track. This plan consists of a total of about 1200 calories daily.

Below is a table to reference throughout for temperature conversions.

| Gas | °F | °C | Fan |
|-----|-----|-----|-----|
| 1 | 275 | 140 | 120 |
| 2 | 300 | 150 | 130 |
| 3 | 325 | 170 | 150 |
| 4 | 350 | 180 | 160 |
| 5 | 375 | 190 | 170 |
| 6 | 400 | 200 | 180 |
| 7 | 425 | 220 | 200 |
| 8 | 450 | 230 | 210 |
| 9 | 475 | 240 | 220 |

## DAY ONE

**Breakfast: Muffin-Tin Quiches with Smoked Cheddar and Potato** (238 calories)

**Ingredients** (6 portions)

- 2 tablespoon extra virgin olive oil
- 1 ½ cups finely diced red-skinned potatoes
- 1 cup red onion
- ¾ teaspoon salt,
- 8 large eggs, divided
- 1 cup smoked Cheddar cheese
- ½ cup low-fat milk
- ½ teaspoon ground black pepper
- 1 ½ cups chopped fresh spinach

Preparation time- 30m. Ready in- 1 hour.

**How to Prepare**

1. Preheat oven to 325°F (160°C). Coat with cooking spray on a 12-cup muffin tin.

2. Heat up oil on a medium heat in a large skillet. Add onions, potatoes and ¼ teaspoon salt and cook, stirring, for about 5 minutes, until the potatoes are just tender. Remove from heat and allow to cool for 5 minutes.

3. In a large bowl, whisk together eggs, cheese, milk, pepper and the remaining ½ teaspoon salt. Stir spinach and potatoes into the mixture. Divide the mixture of quiches into the prepared muffin cups.

4. Bake for about 25 minutes, until firm to the touch. Let stand in the tin for 5 minutes before removing.

5. To save time: cover in plastic individually and refrigerate for up to 3 days or freeze for up to 1 month. Remove plastic to reheat, wrap in a paper towel and microwave for 30 to 60 seconds on high.

**Morning snack:** 1 cup sliced cucumber accompanied with a squeeze of lemon juice and salt and also pepper to taste (16 calories).

**Lunch: Stuffed Sweet Potato with Hummus Dressing** (472 calories).

## Ingredients

- 1 big sweet potato, scrubbed
- ¾ cup chopped kale
- 1 cup black canned beans, rinsed
- ¼ cup hummus
- 2 tablespoons water

## How to Prepare

1. Prick sweet potato with a fork all over. Microwave on high for 7 to 10 minutes, until cooked through.

2. Meanwhile, wash the kale and drain. Layer in a medium saucepan; cover over medium-high heat and cook until wilted, stirring once or twice. Add beans; if the ingredients begin sticking to the pot, add a spoonful or two of water. Continue to cook, uncovered, stir occasionally, for 1 to 2 minutes, until the mixture is steaming.

3. Break open the sweet potato and cover with mixture of kale and beans. Combine the hummus in a small dish with 2 tablespoons of water to create a dressing. Add extra water to achieve

desired consistency as needed. Drizzle the hummus dressing over the stuffed sweet potato.

**Evening snack:** 1 plum (30 calories)

**Dinner: Roasted Root Vegetables and Green over Spiced Lentils** (453 calories).

## Ingredients

- Lentils
- 1 ½ cup water
- ½ cup black beluga lentils or French green lentils
- 1 teaspoon garlic powder
- ½ teaspoon ground coriander
- ½ teaspoon ground cumin
- ¼teaspoon ground allspice
- ¼ teaspoon kosher salt
- 2 teaspoon lemon juice
- 1 teaspoon extra virgin olive oil for the vegetables
- 1 tablespoon extra virgin olive oil
- 1 clove of garlic
- 1 ½ cup roasted root vegetables

## How to Prepare

1. To prepare lentils: Combine water, lentils, garlic powder, ½ teaspoon coriander, cumin, allspice, ¼ teaspoon salt and sumac (if using) in a medium pot. Bring to a boil

2. Reduce heat to keep it simmering, cover and cook until tender for 25-30 minutes.

3. Uncover and continue to boil until the liquid reduces slowly (about 5 minutes longer). Drain and wash. Stir in lemon juice and 1 tablespoon of olive oil.

4. In the meantime, vegetables should be prepared: Heat oil in a large skillet over medium heat. Add the garlic and cook, until fragrant, for 1-2 minutes. Remove the roasted vegetables and cook for 2-4 minutes, stirring often until finished. Stir in the kale (or beet greens) and cook until just wilted for 2-3 minutes. Stir in coriander, pepper and salt.

5. Serve the lentils over the vegetables, and cover with tahini (or yogurt). Garnish over spiced lentils with parsley and orange, if desired.

> Daily total nutritional analysis: 1209 calories, 45 grams fat, 157 grams carbohydrate, 39 grams fiber, 54 grams protein, 1622 mg sodium.

## DAY TWO

**Breakfast: Creamy Blueberry-Pecan Overnight Oatmeal** (291 calories).

**Ingredients**

- ½ cup old-fashioned rolled oats
- ½ cup water Pinch of salt
- ½ cup blueberries, fresh or frozen, thawed
- 2 tablespoon non-fat Greek yogurt
- 1 tablespoon toasted pecans
- 2 teaspoon pure maple syrup

**How to Prepare**

Mix oats, water and salt in a container or bowl. Cover, and cool overnight. Heat up if needed in the morning, and top with blueberries, milk, pecans, and syrup.

**Amount:** 1 serving

**Morning snack:** ½ cup raspberries (32 calories).

**Lunch: Roasted Vegetables and Quinoa Salad** (351 calories).

**Ingredients**

- 200 g quinoa
- 3 tablespoon olive oil
- 1 red onion, peeled but left whole, then cut into 1cm thick round slices 2 peppers, red, yellow or mixture, preferred and cut into chunky long wedges
- 200g baby courgette, halved lengthways
- 3 garlic cloves, unpeeled zest and juice
- 1 lemon
- Pinch of sugar
- Small pack of flat-leaf parsley, roughly chopped
- 200g feta cheese

**How to Prepare**

1. Cook the quinoa following the instructions given on the pack.

2. In the meantime, heat oven to 180/200°C, Gas 6. Throw the onion and peppers on a roasting tray with 1 tablespoon of oil and season, then roast for 15 minutes.

3. Throw the courgettes and garlic together with the rest of the veg and roast for another 15 minutes.

4. Squeeze the roasted garlic cloves out of their skins, and mix with some seasoning. Add the remaining oil, lemon juice and zest, then add sugar to taste. Drizzle over the quinoa and toss the roasted vegetables and the parsley together. Crumble over the feta, throw on and serve.

Amount: 1 serving

**Evening snack:** ½ cup sliced cucumber with pepper and a pinch of salt (8 calories).

**Dinner: One-skillet Salmon with Fennel and Sun-Dried Tomato Couscous** (543 calories).

## Ingredients

- 1 lemon
- 1 ¼ pounds of salmon, skinned and cut into 4 servings
- ¼ teaspoon salt
- ¼ teaspoon ground pepper
- 4 tablespoons sun-dried tomato pesto, divided
- 2 tablespoon extra virgin olive oil, divided
- 2 medium fennel bulbs, cut into 1/2 inch wedges; fronds reserved
- 1 cup Israeli couscous
- 3 scallions of whole wheat, sliced
- 1 ½ cups low-sodium chicken broth
- ¼ cup green olives

## How to Prepare

1. Cut the lemon out into eight slices. Dress salmon with salt and pepper and spread on each piece 1 ½ teaspoons of pesto.

2. Heat 1 tablespoon oil in a large skillet over medium-high heat. Add half the fennel; cook until brown on the bottom, 2 to 3 minutes. Transfer to a plate.

3. Reduce heat to medium and repeat with the remaining 1 tablespoon oil and fennel. Transfer to the plate. Add couscous and scallions to the pan; cook, stirring frequently, until the couscous is lightly toasted, 1 to 2 minutes.

4. Stir in broth, olives, pine nuts, garlic, the reserved lemon zest and the remaining 2 tablespoons pesto.

5. Nestle the fennel into the couscous and the salmon. Finish the salmon with slices of lemon. Reduce heat to low-medium, cover and cook for 10 to 14 minutes until salmon is cooked through and the couscous is tender. When needed, garnish with fennel fronds.

Amount: 4 serving

Daily total nutritional analysis: 1225 calories, 27 grams fiber, 59 grams protein, 51 grams fat, 143 grams carbohydrate, 1130 mg sodium.

## DAY THREE

**Breakfast: Everything Bagel Avocado Toast alongside one of 1 hard-boiled egg** (250 calories).

**Ingredients**

- 1 slice of bread
- ¼ avocado
- 1 tablespoon cream cheese
- 1–2 teaspoon all bagel seasoning

**How to Prepare**

Cover the toasted bread with the cream cheese. Fill with avocado and bagel seasoning all over. Love it!

Amount: 1 serving

**Morning snack:** 1 cup raspberries (64 calories).

**Lunch: Roasted Vegetables and Quinoa Salad** (351 calories).

**Ingredients**

- A bunch of baby beetroot scrubbed, and leaves removed
- 3 small sweet potatoes about 1 lb., peeled and cut into 1" pieces.
- A bunch of baby carrots scrubbed and leaves removed
- 1 medium red onion peeled and cut into 8 pieces
- 10 baby yellow squash about ¼lb., halved
- 1 red pepper cut into 1" pieces
- Olive oil for roasting
- Salt & pepper

For quinoa base

- 1 cup quinoa
- 5 - 6 tablespoons chopped herbs I used parsley, basil and chives
- ¼cup lemon juice
- ¼ cup olive oil
- Salt & pepper

## How to Prepare

1. To roast the vegetables, preheat the oven to 390F

2. Place the beetroot in a large sheet of foil in the middle. Drizzle with olive oil, season with salt and pepper and scrunch the foil to put the beetroot on top. Put in the oven.

3. Add olive oil, salt & pepper to the sweet potato, red onion, carrots, baby squash and red pepper (at different time increments as shown below). Spread over a baking tray and put in the oven.

4. Cook the beetroot for about 45 minutes, or until the beetroot is easily perforated by a skewer. To allow the beetroot to cool slightly, remove from the oven and open the foil packet. Slip the skins off the beetroot when it is cool enough to handle and cut them into pieces. Then put it back in the oven

5. Meanwhile, cook the remaining vegetables until lightly browned and softened. Sweet potato-45 minutes, baby carrots-30 minutes, red onion-30 minutes, baby squash-25 minutes, red pepper-20 minutes.

6. Once happy all the vegetables are roasted, remove the vegetables from the oven. Certain vegetable parts can cook faster than others, so if possible, remove these individually during the cooking time to prevent overcooking.

## For the quinoa base

1. Cook the quinoa according to packet directions while the vegetables are roasting.

2. In a small bowl, mix the lemon juice and the olive oil. Season with salt and pepper, and then whisk in. Put aside.

3. Place the cooked quinoa in a large bowl with the chopped herbs.

4. Season with salt and pepper and swirl the herbs through the quinoa gently.

5. Pour the lemon dressing over the vegetables then toss them into quinoa mix. Serve warm.

Amount: 1 serving

**Evening snack:** 5 oz. non-fat plain Greek yogurt (84 calories).

**Dinner: Mediterranean Chickpea Quinoa Bowl** (479 calories).

## Ingredients

- 1 (7 oz.) jar roasted red peppers, rinsed
- ¼ cup slivered almonds
- 4 tablespoons extra virgin olive oil, divided
- 1 small clove garlic, minced
- 1 teaspoon paprika
- ½ teaspoon ground cumin
- ¼ teaspoon crushed red pepper (optional)
- 2 cups cooked quinoa (about ½ cup uncooked)
- ¼ cup Kalamata olives, cut
- ¼ cup finely chopped red onion
- 1 (15 oz.) can chickpeas, rinsed
- 1 cup diced cucumber
- ¼ cup crumbled feta cheese
- 2 tablespoons finely chopped fresh parsley

## How to Prepare

1. Place peppers, almonds, 2 tablespoons of oil, garlic, paprika, cumin and crushed red pepper in a food processor. Purée until smooth.

2. In a small bowl, combine the quinoa, olives, red onion and the remaining 2 tablespoons of oil.

3. Divide the quinoa mixture into 4 bowls and top with equal amounts of chickpea, cucumber, and red pepper sauce for serving. Sprinkle with parsley and a feta.

Amount: 1 serving

**Meal-prep Tip***:* Thaw the **Slow-cooker Pasta e Fagioli Soup Freezer Pack** inside the fridge overnight. Put in the cooker by morning so it is ready in time for dinner.

Daily total nutritional analysis: 1227 calories, 127 carbohydrates, 30 grams fiber, 50 grams protein, 30 grams fiber, 59 grams fat, 1390 mg sodium.

## DAY FOUR

**Breakfast: Muesli with Raspberries** (278 calories).

**Ingredients**

- ⅓ cup muesli
- 1 cup raspberries
- ¾ cup low fat milk

**How to Prepare**

Top muesli with raspberries and serve with milk.

**Amount:** 1 serving

**Morning snack:** 1 large peach (68 calories).

**Lunch: Roasted Veggie and Quinoa Salad** (351 calories)

**Ingredients:**

- ½ cup zucchini (75g),
- ½ cup cubed sweet potato (100g),
- 1 cup cubed cherry tomato (200g),
- ½ red onion,
- ½ cup diced corn (85g),
- ½ fresh canned lemon, for juice
- 4 tablespoon olive oil,
- 1 teaspoon garlic salt, to taste pepper,
- 4 cups quinoa (680g),
- 1 tablespoon apple cider vinegar
- ¼ cup fresh parsley (10g), chopped

**How to Prepare**

1. Preheat the oven to 350°F (180°C)

2. Line a baking sheet with parchment paper then fill the baking sheet with the zucchini, sweet potatoes, tomatoes, cabbage, and corn.

3. Add the lemon juice and 2 tablespoons of olive oil, then season with salt and pepper. Toss to coat the vegetables uniformly, keeping them apart on the pan.

4. Roast for 15-20 minutes, or tender when stabbed with a fork.

5. Move the roasted vegetables into a big bowl, then add the quinoa.

6. Mix the remaining 2 tablespoons of olive oil and apple cider vinegar together in a small bowl. Garnish the vegetables and quinoa, then toss to coat.

Garnish with parsley. Enjoy!

Amount: 4 serving

**Evening snack:** 1 plum (30 calories)

**Dinner: Slow-Cooker Pasta e Fagioli Soup Freezer Pack** (457 calories)

**Ingredients**

- 2 cups chopped onions
- 1 cup chopped carrots
- 1 cup chopped celery
- 1 pound cooked Meal-Prep Sheet-Pan Chicken Thighs
- 4 cups cooked whole-wheat rotini pasta
- 6 cups reduced-sodium chicken broth
- 4 teaspoons dried Italian seasoning
- ¼ teaspoon salt
- 4 cups baby spinach (½ of a 5 oz. box)
- 4 tablespoons chopped fresh basil, divided (optional)
- 2 tablespoons best-quality extra virgin olive oil
- ½ cup grated Parmigiano-Reggiano cheese

**How to Prepare**

1. Place cooled chicken in one container, and cooked pasta in another.

2. Seal all bags and freeze for a period of 5 days.

3. Defrost the sacks overnight in the refrigerator before continuing.

4. Transfer the vegetable mixture to a large slow cooker. Add broth, Italian seasoning and salt. Cover and cook on Low for 7 ¼ hours.

5. Add beans, spinach, 2 tablespoons basil, if using, and the chicken and pasta defrosted. Cook for 45 minutes. Ladle the soup into bowls. Drizzle a little oil into each bowl and, if needed, top with cheese and the remaining 2 tablespoons of basil.

Amount: 6 serving

Day-to-day total nutritional analysis: 1193 calories, 158 grams carbohydrate, 44 grams fat, 59 grams protein, 33 grams fiber, 1116 mg sodium.

## DAY FIVE

**Breakfast: Everything Bagel Avocado Toast** alongside a dish of 1 hard-boiled egg. (250 calories)

### Ingredients

- 1 slice of bread
- ¼ avocado
- 1 tablespoon cream cheese
- 1–2 teaspoon all bagel seasoning

### How to Prepare

Cover the toasted bread with the cream cheese. Fill with avocado and bagel seasoning all over. Love it!

Amount: 1 serving

**Lunch:** 1 serving **Roasted Veggie and Quinoa Salad** (351 calories)

### Ingredients

- ½ cup zucchini (75g),

- ½ cup cubed sweet potato (100g),
- 1 cup cubed cherry tomato (200g),
- ½ red onion,
- ½ cup diced corn (85g),
- ½ fresh or canned lemon, for juice
- 4 tablespoons olive oil,
- 1 teaspoon garlic salt, to taste pepper,
- 4 cups quinoa (680g),
- 1 tablespoon apple cider vinegar
- ¼ cup fresh parsley (10g), chopped

**How to Prepare**

1. Preheat the oven to 350°F (180°C)

2. Line a baking sheet with parchment paper then fill the baking sheet with the zucchini, sweet potatoes, tomatoes, cabbage, and corn.

3. Add the lemon juice and 2 tablespoons of olive oil, then season with salt and pepper. Toss to coat the vegetables uniformly, keeping them apart on the pan.

4. Roast for 15-20 minutes, or tender when stabbed with a fork.

5. Move the roasted vegetables into a big bowl, then add the quinoa.

6. Mix the remaining 2 tablespoons of olive oil and apple cider vinegar together in a small bowl. Garnish the vegetables and quinoa, then toss to coat.

Garnish with parsley. Enjoy!

Amount: 4 serving

**Evening snack:** 1 cup non-fat plain Greek yogurt with 1 tablespoon of chopped (cut up) walnuts (181 calories)

**Dinner: Noodle Eggplant Lasagna** with 2 cups mixed greens topped with 1 tablespoon **Herb Vinaigrette** (364 calories)

## Ingredients

- 2 large eggplants (total 2½-3 pounds), sliced lengthwise into ¼ inch thick slices
- 1 tablespoon extra virgin olive oil
- 12 oz. of lean ground beef
- 1 cup chopped onion
- 2 cloves of garlic, chopped
- 1 (28 oz.) crushed tomatoes
- ¼ cup dry red wine 1 teaspoon dried basil
- 1 teaspoon dried oregano
- ¾ teaspoon salt
- ¼ teaspoon ground pepper
- 1½ cup part-skim ricotta cheese
- 1 large egg, lightly beaten
- 1 cup shredded part-skim mozzarella cheese, divided
- Chopped fresh basil for garnish

## How to Prepare

1. Coat 2 large trays with baking sheets

2. Arrange eggplant slices on prepared pans in a single layer. Roast for 15 to 20 minutes, until tender.

3. Meanwhile, heat up oil over a medium-high heat in a large skillet. Add beef and onion; cook, stir and chop with a wooden spoon for 6 to 8 minutes, until browned. Add the garlic and cook for 1 minute. Add the tomatoes, wine, basil, oregano, salt and pepper. Reduce heat to low-medium, and cook for about more 10 minutes, stirring occasionally until thickened.

4. Mix egg and ricotta in a small bowl.

5. In a 9x13 inch baking dish, spread around 1 cup the sauce. Arrange ¼ slices of eggplant over the tomato sauce. Dollop the ricotta mixture on about ⅓ cup, and scatter with ¼ cup mozzarella.

6. Create another layer of the eggplant slices with another ¼, this time grouping them crosswise to the first one. Finish with 1 cup sauce, dollop with ⅓ cup ricotta and sprinkle with ¼ cup mozzarella. Repeat with the remaining ingredients to create 2 more layers.

7. Bake the lasagna, uncovered, for 30 to 40 minutes, until the sauce bubbles around its edges. Let stand before serving for 10–20 minutes. If needed, garnish with fresh basil.

Day-to-day total nutritional analysis: 1206 calories, 58 grams fat, 103 grams carbohydrates, 31 grams fiber, 1272 mg sodium, 74 grams protein.

## DAY SIX

**Breakfast:** 1 serving **Muesli with Raspberries** (287 calories)

**Ingredients**

- 1/3 cup muesli
- 1 cup raspberries
- ¾ cup low fat milk

**How to Prepare**

Top muesli with raspberries and serve with milk.

**Morning snack:** 1 big peach (68 calories)

**Lunch: Noodle Eggplant Lasagna** (301 calories)

**Ingredients**

- 2 large eggplants (total 2½ -3 pounds), sliced lengthwise into ¼ inch thick slices
- 1 tablespoon extra virgin olive oil
- 12 oz. of lean ground beef
- 1 cup chopped onion
- 2 cloves of garlic, chopped
- 1 (28 oz.) crushed tomatoes
- ¼ cup dry red wine 1 teaspoon dried basil
- 1 teaspoon dried oregano
- ¾ teaspoon salt
- ¼ teaspoon ground pepper
- 1 ½ cup part-skim ricotta cheese
- 1 big egg, lightly beaten
- 1 cup shredded part-skim mozzarella cheese, divided
- Chopped fresh basil for garnish

**How to Prepare**

1. Coat 2 large trays with baking sheets

2. Arrange eggplant slices on prepared pans in a single layer. Roast for 15 to 20 minutes, until tender.

3. Meanwhile, heat up oil over a medium-high heat in a large skillet. Add beef and onion; cook, stir and chop with a wooden spoon for 6 to 8 minutes, until browned. Add the garlic and cook for 1 minute. Add the tomatoes, wine, basil, oregano, salt and pepper. Reduce heat to low-medium, and cook for about more 10 minutes, stirring occasionally until thickened.

4. Mix egg and ricotta in a small bowl.

5. In a 9x13 inch baking dish, spread around 1 cup the sauce. Arrange ¼ slices of eggplant over the tomato sauce. Dollop the ricotta mixture on about ⅓ cup, and scatter with ¼ cup mozzarella.

6. Create another layer of the eggplant slices with another ¼ mozzarella, this time grouping them crosswise to the first one. Finish with 1 cup sauce, dollop with ⅓ cup ricotta and sprinkle with ¼

cup mozzarella. Repeat with the remaining ingredients to create 2 more layers.

7. Bake the lasagna, uncovered, for 30 to 40 minutes, until the sauce bubbles around its edges. Let stand before serving for 10–20 minutes. If needed, garnish with fresh basil.

**Evening snack:** 1 cup sliced red bell pepper with 3 tablespoon s of hummus (106 calories)

## Dinner: Slow-Cooker Mediterranean Chicken and Chickpea Soup (446 calories)

### Ingredients

- 1 ½ cups dried chickpeas, soaked overnight
- 4 cups water
- 1 large yellow onion, finely chopped
- 1 (15 oz.) can no-salt-added diced tomatoes, preferably fire-roasted
- 2 tablespoons tomato paste
- 4 cloves garlic, finely chopped
- 1 bay leaf
- 4 teaspoons ground cumin
- 4 teaspoons paprika
- ¼ teaspoon cayenne pepper
- ¼ teaspoon ground pepper
- 2 pounds chicken thighs, skin removed, trimmed
- 1 (14 oz.) can artichoke hearts, drained and quartered
- ¼ cup halved pitted oil-cured olives
- ½ teaspoon salt
- ¼ cup chopped fresh parsley or cilantro

### How to Prepare

1. Drain chickpeas and place in a 6-quart or larger slow cooker.

2. Add water, onion, tomatoes and their juice (up to 4 cups worth), tomato paste, garlic, bay leaf, cumin, paprika, cayenne and ground pepper; stir to combine.

3. Stir in chicken.

4. Cover and cook for 8 hours on low or 4 hours on high.

5. Place the chicken on a clean cutting board and allow to cool slightly. Dispose of the bay leaf. Remove the slow cooker with the artichokes, olives and salt, and stir to combine. Shred the bird and discard the bones. Cut the chicken over the broth. Serve with parsley (or cilantro) on top.

Amount: 1 serving

Daily total nutritional analysis: 1209 calories, 1431 mg sodium, 77 grams protein, 143 grams carbohydrates, 38 grams fiber, 40 grams fat.

## DAY SEVEN

**Breakfast: Everything Bagel Avocado Toast** plus a side dish of 1 hard-boiled egg- Check above for Recipe

**Morning snack:** ½ cup raspberries (31 calories)

**Lunch: Slow-Cooker Mediterranean Chicken and Chickpea Soup** (446 calories)

**Ingredients**

- 1 ½ cups dried chickpeas, soaked overnight
- 4 cups water
- 1 large yellow onion, finely chopped
- 1 (15 oz.) can of no-salt-added diced tomatoes, preferably fire-roasted
- 2 tablespoon tomato paste

- 4 cloves of garlic, finely chopped
- 1 bay leaf
- 4 teaspoons ground cumin
- 4 teaspoons paprika
- ¼ teaspoon cayenne pepper
- ¼ teaspoon ground pepper
- 2 pounds chicken thighs, skin removed, trimmed
- 1 (14 oz.) can of artichoke hearts, drained and quartered
- ¼ cup halved pitted oil-cured olives
- ½ teaspoon salt
- ¼ cup chopped fresh parsley or cilantro

**How to Prepare**

1. Drain chickpeas and place in a 6-quart or larger slow cooker.

2. Add water, onion, tomatoes and their juice (up to 4 cups worth), tomato paste, garlic, bay leaf, cumin, paprika, cayenne and ground pepper; stir to combine. Stir in chicken.

3. Cover and cook for 8 hours on low or 4 hours on high.

4. Place the chicken on a clean cutting board and allow to cool slightly. Dispose of the bay leaf. Remove the slow cooker with the artichokes, olives and salt, and stir to combine. Shred the bird and discard the bones. Cut the chicken over the broth. Serve with parsley (or cilantro) on top

**Evening snack:** ½ sliced cucumber with pepper and a pinch of salt.

**Dinner:** one serving **One-Pot Greek Pasta** (487 calories)

**Ingredients**

- 2 tablespoon olive oil
- 3 links of cooked chicken sausage (9 oz.), sliced into rounds
- 1 cup diced onion (see Tip)

- 1 clove of garlic, minced
- 1 (8 oz.) can of no-salt-added tomato sauce
- 4 cups lightly packed baby spinach (½ of a 5 oz. box)
- 6 cups cooked whole-wheat rotini pasta
- ¼ cup chopped pitted Kalamata olives
- ½ cup finely crumbled feta cheese
- ¼ cup chopped fresh basil (optional)

**How to Prepare**

1. Heat oil in a large straight-sided skillet over medium-high heat. Add sausage, onion and garlic; cook, stirring constantly, for 4 to 6 minutes, until the onion starts to brown.

2. Add tomato sauce, spinach, pasta and olives; cook for 3 to 5 minutes, stirring frequently, until bubbling hot and wilting the spinach. If required, add 1 to 2 tablespoons of water to keep the pasta from sticking. Apply feta and basil, if used.

## DAY EIGHT

**Breakfast: Creamy Blueberry-Pecan Overnight Oatmeal** (291 calories)

**Ingredients**

- ½ cup old-fashioned rolled oats
- ½ cup water
- Pinch of salt
- ½ cup blueberries, fresh or frozen, thawed
- 2 tablespoon non-fat plain Greek yogurt
- 1 tablespoon toasted chopped pecans
- 2 teaspoon pure maple syrup

**How to Prepare**

In a jar or cup, mix the oats, water, and salt. Cover, and cool overnight. Heat up if needed in the morning, and top with blueberries, milk, pecans, and syrup.

**Morning snack:** 1 cup blackberries (62 calories)

**Lunch: Slow-Cooker Mediterranean Chicken and Chickpea Soup** (446 calories) - Check above for Recipe

**Evening snack:** 1 plum (30 calories)

**Dinner: Summer Shrimp Salad** plus 2 cups mixed greens topped with one tablespoon **Parsley-Lemon Vinaigrette** (39 calories)

**Ingredients**

- 1 ¼ pounds of raw shrimp (21-25 count), peeled and deveined
- ¼ cup extra virgin olive oil
- 10 sprigs of fresh thyme
- 4 cloves of garlic, crushed

41

- ¼ teaspoon salt
- ¼ teaspoon ground pepper
- ¼ cup lemon juice
- 1 medium English cucumber, diced
- 3 large heirloom tomatoes, chopped
- ½ cup chopped fresh basil, plus more for garnish

**How to Prepare**

1. Preheat oven to 350°F (180°C).

2. Toss the shrimp on a rimmed baking sheet with butter, thyme and garlic. Sprinkle with pepper and salt. Bake for 8 to 10 minutes, until the shrimp are pink and strong.

3. Move the shrimp (discard thyme and garlic) to a large bowl. Add lemon juice to cover and mix. Stir gently in cucumber, basil and tomatoes. Put the shrimp and vegetables in a bowl for serving. Serve with any dressing left in the cup, and garnish, if needed, with more basil.

Daily total nutritional analysis: 1224 calories, 49 grams fat, 77 grams protein, 1420 mg sodium, 127 grams carbohydrates, 31 grams fiber.

## DAY NINE

**Breakfast: Muesli with Raspberries** (287 calories) - Check above for Recipe

**Morning snack:** ½ cup sliced cucumbers with pepper and a pinch of salt (8 calories)

**Lunch: Vegan Superfood Buddha Bowls** (381 calories)

**Ingredients**

- 1 (8 oz.) pouch microwavable quinoa
- ½ cup hummus

- 2 tablespoon lemon juice
- 1 (5 oz.) package of baby kale
- 1 (8 oz.) package of refrigerated cooked whole baby beets, sliced (or 2 cups from salad bar)
- 1 cup frozen shelled edamame, thawed
- 1 medium avocado, sliced
- ¼ cup unsalted, toasted sunflower seeds

## How to Prepare

1. Prepare quinoa as guided in the package; set aside to cool.

2. Combine the lemon juice and hummus in a small bowl. Thin with water, to the desired consistency of dressing. Divide and refrigerate the dressing into 4 small condiment containers with lids.

3. Divide the baby kale into 4 single-serving lids containers. Finish each one with ½ cup quinoa, ½ cup beets, ¼ cup edamame and 1 sunflower seed tablespoon.

4. When you're ready to eat, top with ¼ avocado and the dressing with hummus.

**Evening snack:** ½ cup sliced red bell pepper (14 calories)

**Dinner: Lemon Tahini Couscous with Chicken and Vegetables** (528 calories)

## Ingredients

- 1 cup whole-wheat pearl couscous
- ¼ cup tahini
- ¼ cup water
- 2 teaspoon lemon zest
- 2 tablespoon lemon juice
- 2 tablespoon olive oil, divided
- ½ teaspoon salt
- ¼ teaspoon ground pepper

- ¼ teaspoon crushed red pepper
- 1 clove of garlic, minced
- 2 cups sliced mushrooms (½ of a 10 oz. package)
- ½ medium red bell pepper, chopped
- 4 cups coleslaw mix (½ of a 12 to 14 oz. package)
- 4 cups baby spinach (½ of a 5 oz. bag)
- 12 oz. cooked chicken breast, chopped (about 2½ cups)
- ¼ cup toasted sliced almonds
- ¼ cup crumbled reduced-fat feta cheese
- 1 tablespoon chopped fresh parsley
- 1 lemon, cut into wedges (optional)

**How to Prepare**

1. Cook the couscous in a medium saucepan as instructed by the packet. Fluff with a fork and set it aside.

2. In the meantime, whisk the tahini, tea, 1 tablespoon of oil and lemon juice in a small bowl. Then add in the butter, salt, pepper and crushed red pepper, until well mixed; set aside.

3. Steam the remaining 1 tablespoon of oil over medium-high heat in a big, non-stick skillet. Add the garlic and cook for about 30 seconds, until it is fragrant. Add mushrooms and bell pepper; cook for about 3 minutes, until the mushrooms release their liquid.

4. Add coleslaw mixture and spinach; continue cooking, stirring, for about 2 minutes, until the spinach wilts. Add the chicken, the couscous and the tahini sauce; cook for 2 to 4 minutes until warm.

5. Sprinkle with almonds, feta, lemon zest and parsley. When needed serve with lemon wedges.

Daily total nutritional analysis: 1219 calories, 983 mg sodium, 70 grams protein, 141 grams carbohydrate, 49 grams fat, 36 grams fiber.

## DAY TEN

**Breakfast: Muffin-Tin Quiches with Smoked Cheddar and Potato** (238 calories)

### Ingredients

- 2 tablespoon extra virgin olive oil
- 1 ½ cups finely diced red-skinned potatoes
- 1 cup diced red onion
- ¾ teaspoon salt, divided
- 8 large eggs
- 1 cup shredded smoked Cheddar cheese
- ½ cup low-fat milk
- ½ teaspoon ground black pepper
- 1 ½ cups chopped fresh spinach

### How to Prepare

1. Preheat oven to 325°F (160°C). Coat with cooking spray on a 12-cup muffin tin.

2. Heat up oil over medium heat in a large skillet. Add onions, potatoes and ¼ teaspoon salt and cook, stirring for about 5 minutes, until the potatoes are just done. Remove from heat and allow to cool for 5 minutes.

3. In a large bowl, whisk together eggs, cheese, milk, pepper and the remaining ½ teaspoon of salt. Stir into the mixture the spinach and potatoes. Divide the mixture of quiches into the prepared muffin cups.

4. Bake for about 25 minutes, until firm to the touch. Let stand from the tin for 5 minutes before removing.

**Morning snack:** ½ cup raspberries (32 calories)

**Lunch: Vegan Superfood Buddha Bowl** (381 calories) - Check above for Recipe

**Evening snack:** ½ cup blackberries (31 calories)

**Dinner:** Take 1 serving **Walnut-Rosemary Crusted Salmon** with 1 serving of **Easy Brown Rice Pilaf with Spring Vegetables** (538 calories)

---

Daily total nutritional analysis: 1219 calories,1273 mg sodium, 65 grams protein, 120 grams carbohydrates, 56 grams fat, 30 grams fiber.

---

## DAY ELEVEN

**Breakfast: Berry-Mint Kefir Smoothie** (274 calories)

**Ingredients**

- 1 cup low-fat plain kefir (see Tip)
- 1 cup frozen mixed berries
- ¼ cup orange juice
- 1-2 tablespoons fresh mint
- 1 tablespoon honey

**How to Prepare**

In a blender, mix kefir, berries, tea, taste mint and honey. Work through until smooth. (The smoothies should be kept in the fridge for up to 1 day or in the freezer for up to 3 months.)

**Morning snack:** 1 plum (30 calories)

**Lunch: Vegan Superfood Buddha Bowl** (381 calories) - Check above for Recipe

**Evening snack:** ½ cup non-fat plain Greek yogurt (66 calories)

**Dinner: Farfalle with Tuna, Lemon and Fennel** with 2 cups mixed greens and 1 tablespoon **Parsley-Lemon Vinaigrette** (460 calories)

**Ingredients**

- 6 oz. dried whole grain farfalle (bow tie) pasta

- 1 (5 oz.) canned solid white tuna (packed in oil)
- Olive oil (optional)
- 1 cup fennel, thinly sliced (1 medium bulb)
- 2 cloves garlic, minced
- ½ teaspoon crushed red pepper
- ¼ teaspoon salt
- 2 (14.5 oz.) cans no-salt-added diced tomatoes, undrained
- 2 tablespoons snipped fresh Italian (flat leaf) parsley
- 1 teaspoon lemon peel, finely shredded

**How to Prepare**

1. Cook pasta as indicated by box, omitting salt; drain. Return the pasta to the pan; cover and keep warm. While cooking the pasta, remove the excess oil from the tuna. Save enough olive oil if necessary, to weigh a minimum of 3 cubic tablespoons. Flake the tuna out of the tin using a fork.

2. Heat the 3 tablespoons of reserved oil in a medium saucepan over medium heat. Attach the fennel; cook, stirring occasionally for 3 minutes. Add garlic, crushed red pepper, and salt; cook and stir for about 1 minute, or until the garlic is golden.

3. Stir tomatoes in. Bring them to boil; reduce heat. Simmer for 5 to 6 minutes, uncovered, or until mixture starts to thicken. Stir in the tuna; cook, open, about 1 more minute or until the tuna is heated through.

4. Pour the tuna over pasta; gently stir to combine. Sprinkle with parsley and lemon peel to each serving.

Daily total nutritional analysis: 1211 calories, 910 mg sodium, 59 grams protein, 34 grams fiber, 155 grams carbohydrates, 45 grams fiber.

## DAY TWELVE

**Breakfast: Muffin-Tin Quiches with Smoked Cheddar and Potato** (238 calories) - Check above for Recipe

**Morning snack:** 1 plum (30 calories)

**Lunch: Vegan Superfood Buddha Bowls** (381 calories) - Check above for recipe

**Evening snack:** 5 oz. non-fat plain Greek yogurt with ¼ cup blueberries (105 calories)

**Dinner: Cilantro Bean Burgers with Creamy Avocado-Lime Slaw** plus 2 cups mixed greens and 1 tablespoon **Parsley-Lemon Vinaigrette** (472 calories)

Ingredients

- 1 (15 oz.) can no-salt-added black beans, rinsed
- 2 cloves garlic, minced, divided
- ½ teaspoon ground cumin
- ½ teaspoon salt, divided
- ⅛ teaspoon ground pepper
- ¼ cup crushed tortilla chips or panko breadcrumbs
- ¼ cup quick-cooking oats
- 2 tablespoons toasted pumpkin seeds, chopped
- 2 tablespoons chopped fresh cilantro plus ½ cup, divided
- 1 large egg, lightly beaten
- ¼ cup low-fat plain Greek yogurt
- ½ avocado
- 1 teaspoon lime zest
- 2 tablespoons lime juice
- 2 tablespoons water
- 4 cups shredded cabbage (green and/or red)
- 2 teaspoons olive oil
- 4 whole-wheat buns, halved and toasted

**How to Prepare**

1. Combine beans, half the garlic, cumin, ¼ teaspoon salt, and pepper in a medium bowl. Mash with a fork until all the beans are smashed. Stir in crushed chips (or panko), oats, pumpkin seeds, 2 tablespoons cilantro, and egg.

2. Divide the mixture into 4 portions, then shape into patties. Place on a plate and refrigerate for 30 minutes before cooking.

3. Meanwhile, combine the remaining ½ cup cilantro, the remaining garlic, yogurt, avocado, lime juice, and water in a blender or food processor. Puree until smooth. Transfer to a large bowl. Stir in lime zest and the remaining ¼ teaspoon salt. Add cabbage and toss to combine.

4. Heat oil in a large nonstick skillet over medium-high heat. Add the patties and cook for 6 minutes. Turn them over, reduce heat to medium, cover and cook until golden brown and warmed through, 5 to 6 minutes more. Serve the burgers on buns, topped with ¼ cup cabbage slaw each. Serve the remaining slaw on the side.

Daily total nutritional analysis: 1226 calories, 1619 mg, 63 grams protein, 56 grams fat, 34 grams fiber, 130 grams carbohydrate.

## DAY THIRTEEN

**Breakfast: Berry-Mint Kefir Smoothies** (274 calories) - Check above for Recipe

**Morning snack:** ⅔ cup raspberries (42 calories)

**Lunch: Mason Jar Power Salad with Chickpeas and Tuna** (430 calories)

**Ingredients**

- 3 cups bite-sized pieces chopped kale
- 2 tablespoons honey-mustard vinaigrette (see associated recipe)
- 2.5 oz. pouch tuna in water
- ½ cup rinsed canned chickpeas
- 1 carrot, peeled and shredded

**How to Prepare**

1. Mix kale and dress in a pot, then move to a 1-quarter mason jar. Fill with the salmon, carrot and chickpeas. Screw the lid onto the container, and cool for up to 2 days.

2. To serve, pour the contents of the jar into a bowl and mix the salad ingredients together with the dressed kale.

**Evening snack:** ⅔ cup blackberries (41 calories)

**Dinner: Roasted Chicken and Winter Squash over Mixed Greens** (415 calories)

**Ingredients**

- 2 ½ pounds delicata or acorn squash
- 3 tablespoons extra virgin olive oil, divided
- 2 tablespoons whole-grain mustard, divided
- 3 cloves garlic, minced
- 1 tablespoon chopped fresh rosemary or 1 teaspoon dried
- 1 teaspoon grated lemon zest
- 2 tablespoons lemon juice, divided
- 1 teaspoon ground pepper, divided
- ½ teaspoon salt, divided
- 1 pound boneless, skinless chicken breast
- 1 tablespoon pure maple syrup
- 1 ½ teaspoons fresh thyme leaves
- 8 cups mixed salad greens
- 4 teaspoons grated Parmesan cheese
- 4 teaspoons salted roasted pumpkin

**How to Prepare**

1. Preheat oven to 425°F (220°C). Coat with the cooking spray on a wide rimmed baking sheet.

2. Lengthwise cut squash in half, and extract seeds. Cut 1 inch slices crosswise.

3. In a large bowl, mix 1 tablespoon of oil, 1½ tablespoons of mustard, garlic, rosemary, lemon zest, ½ tablespoon of lemon juice, ½ teaspoon of pepper and ¼ teaspoon salt. Add chicken and squash to coat and stir. Arrange onto the prepared pan in a single layer.

4. Bake until the squash starts to brown, and the chicken reaches an internal temperature of 165°F (80°C) for 20-22 minutes, without stirring or flipping. Move the chicken onto a clean slice and cutting plate.

5. In a medium bowl, whisk the remaining 2 tablespoons of butter, ½ tablespoon of mustard, 1½ tablespoon of lemon juice, maple syrup, thyme and the remaining ½ teaspoon of pepper and ¼ teaspoon of salt. Add greens to cover, and throw

6. Divide the greens into 4 serving plates. Finish with the seeds for chicken and squash, Parmesan, and pumpkin.

> Daily total nutritional analysis: 1202 calories, 34 grams fiber, 72 grams protein, 142 grams carbohydrates, 42 grams fat, 1192 mg sodium

## DAY FOURTEEN

**Breakfast: Berry-Mint Kefir Smoothies** (274 calories) - Check above for Recipe

**Morning snack:** ½ cup raspberries (32 calories)

**Lunch: Mason Jar Power Salad with Chickpeas and Tuna** (430 calories) - Check above for Recipe

**Evening snack**: ½ cup blackberries (31 calories)

**Dinner: Sweet and Spicy Roasted Salmon with Wild Rice Pilaf** with 2 cups mixed greens and 1 tablespoon **Parsley-Lemon Vinaigrette** (443 calories)

## Ingredients

- 5 skinless salmon fillets, fresh or frozen (1¼ lbs.)
- 2 tablespoons balsamic vinegar
- 1 tablespoon honey
- ¼ teaspoon salt
- ⅛ teaspoon ground pepper
- 1 cup chopped red and/or yellow bell pepper
- ½ to 1 small jalapeño pepper, seeded and finely chopped
- 2 scallions (green parts only), thinly sliced
- ¼ cup chopped fresh Italian parsley
- 2⅔ cups Wild Rice Pilaf

## How to Prepare

1. Thaw salmon, if frozen. Preheat oven to 425°F (220°C). Line a 15x10 inch baking pan with parchment paper. Place the salmon in the prepared pan. Whisk vinegar and honey in a small bowl; drizzle half of the mixture over the salmon. Sprinkle with salt and pepper.

2. Roast the salmon until the thickest part flakes easily, about 15 minutes. Drizzle with the remaining vinegar mixture.

3. Coat a 10 inch non-stick skillet with cooking spray, heat over medium heat. Add bell pepper and jalapeño; cook, stirring frequently, just until tender, 3-5 minutes. Remove from heat. Stir in scallion greens.

4. Top 4 of the salmon fillets with the pepper mixture and parsley. Serve with pilaf. (Refrigerate the remaining salmon for another recipe.)

Daily total nutritional analysis: 1210 calories, 40 grams fat, 1241 mg sodium, 30 grams fiber, 72 grams protein, 145 grams carbohydrates.

# WEEK THREE

## DAY FIFTEEN

**Breakfast: Pineapple Green Smoothie** (297 calories)

**Morning snack:** ¾ cup raspberries (48 calories)

**Lunch: Mediterranean Tuna-Spinach Salad** (375 calories)

**Evening snack:** ¾ cup blackberries (46 calories)

**Dinner: Dijon Salmon with Green Bean Pilaf** (442 calories)

**Ingredients**

- 1¼ pounds wild salmon (see Tip), skinned and cut into 4 portions
- 3 tablespoons extra virgin olive oil, divided
- 1 tablespoon minced garlic
- ¾ teaspoon salt
- 2 tablespoons mayonnaise
- 2 teaspoons whole-grain mustard
- ½ teaspoon ground pepper, divided
- 12 oz. pretrimmed haricots verts or thin green beans, cut into thirds
- 1 small lemon, zested and cut into 4 wedges
- 2 tablespoons pine nuts
- 1 8 oz. package precooked brown rice
- 2 tablespoons water
- Chopped fresh parsley for garnish

**How to Prepare**

1. Preheat oven to 425°F (220°C). Line a baking sheet rimmed with foil or parchment paper.

2. Brush the salmon with 1 spoonful of oil and put them on the prepared baking sheet. Mash the garlic and salt with the side of a chef's knife or a fork into a paste. In a small bowl, mix a meager 1

tablespoon of the garlic paste with mayonnaise, mustard and ¼ teaspoon of pepper. Spread the blend over the water.

3. Roast the salmon with a fork in the thickest part, 6 to 8 minutes per inch thickness, until it flakes easily.

4. In the meantime, heat the remaining 2 tablespoons of oil over medium - high heat in a large skillet. Add green beans, lemon zest, pine nuts, remaining garlic paste and ¼ teaspoon pepper; cook, stirring, for 2-4 minutes until the beans are just tender. Restrain heat to average. Add the rice and water and cook for 2-3 minutes, stirring, until dry.

5. If needed, sprinkle the salmon with parsley and serve with the green bean pilaf and lemon wedges.

> Daily total nutritional analysis: 1209 calories, 53 grams fat, 73 grams protein, 123 grams carbohydrates, 31 grams fiber, 1412 mg sodium.

## DAY SIXTEEN

**Breakfast: Muffin-Tin Quiches with Smoked Cheddar and Potato** (238 calories) - Check above for Recipe

**Morning Snack**: ¾ cup raspberries (48 calories)

**Lunch: Instant Pot White Chicken Chilli Freezer Pack** with a side dish of 2 celery stalks and 3 tablespoon hummuses (346 calories)

**Ingredients**

- 1 medium zucchini, chopped
- 1½ cups frozen corn kernels
- 1 large onion, chopped (about 1⅓ cups)
- 3 cloves garlic, minced
- 2 tablespoons canned diced mild green chiles
- 1 tablespoon chilli powder

- 1¾ teaspoons ground cumin
- 1 teaspoon dried oregano
- ½ teaspoon ground pepper
- ½ teaspoon salt
- 1 pound boneless, skinless chicken breast
- 1¾ cups dry great northern beans
- 4 cups low-sodium chicken broth
- 1½ cups water
- ⅓ cup chopped fresh cilantro, plus more for garnish
- Lime wedges, sour cream and diced avocado (optional)

**How to Prepare**

1. To cook and freeze: In a 64 oz. tub, add zucchini, corn, onion, garlic, chiles, chilli powder, cumin, oregano, pepper, and salt. Pour over the rice, then the beans. Seal and freeze, for up to 3 months, until ready to use.

2. To cook: Let the frozen soup mix stand for 10 minutes at room temperature. Invert the frozen soup mix into a multicooker (beans at the bottom of the pot should be on). Add water and broth. Lock the lid in place and cook for 30 minutes at high pressure. Naturally let the pressure out.

3. Move the chicken and shred it on a cutting board. Put the chicken back into the pot and stir in the coriander. If needed, serve topped with extra cilantro, lime wedges, sour cream and diced avocado.

**Evening Snack:** 2 plums (61 calories)

**Dinner: Chicken and Vegetable Penne with Parsley-Walnut Pesto** (514 calories)

**Ingredients**

- ¾ cup chopped walnuts
- 1 cup lightly packed parsley leaves
- 2 cloves garlic, crushed and peeled

- ½ teaspoon plus ⅛ teaspoon salt
- ⅛ teaspoon ground pepper
- 2 tablespoons olive oil
- ⅓ cup grated Parmesan cheese
- 1½ cups shredded or sliced cooked skinless chicken breast (8 oz.)
- 6 oz. whole-wheat penne or fusilli pasta (1¾ cups)
- 8 oz. green beans, trimmed and halved crosswise (2 cups)
- 2 cups cauliflower florets (8 oz.)

**How to Prepare**

1. Bring a large saucepan of water to boil.

2. Place walnuts in a small bowl and microwave on high for 2-2½ minutes, until fragrant and lightly toasted. (Alternatively, toast the walnuts over medium-low heat in a small dry skillet, stirring constantly, until fragrant, 2- 3 minutes.) Move to the plate and allow to cool. Set aside ¼ cup to top it off.

3. In a food processor, mix the remaining ½ cup walnuts, parsley, garlic, salt, and pepper. Process before grounded nuts. Gradually add oil through the feed pipe with the motor running. Pulse and add Parmesan before blended in. Scrape the pesto in a large saucepan. Stir in chicken.

4. Alternatively, cook the pasta for 4 minutes in boiling water. Add green beans and cauliflower; cover and cook for 5-7 minutes more until the pasta is al dente (still slightly firm) and the vegetables are tender. Scoop out ¾ cup the cooking water before boiling and stir in the pesto-chicken mixture to warm it up slightly. Drain the vegetables and pasta and add to the pesto-chicken mixture. Toss well to coat. Divide between 4 bowls of pasta and finish each serving with 1 tablespoon. Of the Walnuts held.

Daily Total nutritional analysis: 1,206 calories, 75 grams protein, 50 grams fat, 32 grams fiber, 126 grams carbohydrates, 1996 mg sodium.

# DAY SEVENTEEN

**Breakfast: Muffin-Tin Quiches with Smoked Cheddar and Potato** (238 calories) - Check above for Recipe

**Morning snack:** 1 peach (68 calories)

**Lunch: Instant Pot White Chicken Chilli Freezer Pack plus a side of 2 celery stalks and 3 tablespoons of hummus** (346 calories) - Check above for Recipe

**Evening Snack:** ¾ cup blackberries with 6 walnut halves (125 calories)

**Dinner: Greek Turkey Burgers with Spinach, Feta & Tzatziki** with a side of 2 cups mixed greens topped with 1 tablespoon of Basil Vinaigrette (442 calories)

**Ingredients**

- 1 cup frozen chopped spinach, thawed
- 1 pound 93% lean ground turkey
- ½ cup crumbled feta cheese
- ½ teaspoon garlic powder
- ½ teaspoon dried oregano
- ¼ teaspoon salt
- ¼ teaspoon ground pepper
- 4 small hamburger buns, preferably whole-wheat, split
- 4 tablespoons tzatziki
- 12 slices cucumber
- 8 thick rings of red onion (about ¼ inch)

**How to Prepare**

1. Preheat barbecue to medium-high.

2. Squeeze out the remaining spinach moisture. Combine the spinach in a medium bowl with beef, feta, garlic powder, oregano, salt and pepper; mix well. Shape into 4 inch patties.

3. Coat the grill rack with oil. Grill the patties until cooked through, 4-6 minutes per side, and no longer pink in the middle. (An instant read thermometer inserted in the middle should be 165°F/80°C.)

4. Assemble the burgers on the buns, each with 1 tzatziki tablespoon, 3 slices of cucumber and 2 rings of red onion.

Daily total nutritional analysis: 1,219 calories, 78 grams protein, 118 grams carbohydrates, 32 grams fiber, 54 grams fat, 2,205 mg sodium.

## DAY EIGHTEEN

**Breakfast: Muffin-Tin Quiches with Smoked Cheddar and Potato** (238 calories) - Check above for Recipe

**Morning Snack:** 2 plums (61 calories)

**Lunch: Instant Pot White Chicken Chilli Freezer** Pack with a side dish of 2 celery stalks and 3 tablespoons of hummus (346 calories) - Check above for Recipe

**Evening Snack:** 1 large peach (68 calories)

**Dinner: Meal-Prep Falafel Bowls with Tahini Sauce** (500 calories)

**Ingredients**

- 1 (8 oz.) package frozen prepared falafel
- ⅔ cup water
- ½ cup whole-wheat couscous
- 1 (16 oz.) bag steam-in-bag fresh green beans
- ½ cup Tahini Sauce (see associated recipe)
- ¼ cup pitted Kalamata olives
- ¼ cup crumbled feta cheese

**How to Prepare**

1. Prepare falafel as guided by packet; set aside to cool.

2. Bring water in a small saucepan to boil. Remove from heat and pour in couscous. Allow to stand, about 5 minutes, until the liquid is absorbed. Fluffing with a fork; put to the side.

3. Prepare green beans as directed by box.

4. Prepare the sauce for Tahini. Divide and refrigerate among 4 small containers of condiments with lids.

5. Divide the green beans into 4 single-serve lid containers. Finish each with ½ cup couscous, ¼ falafel and 1 tablespoon per feta and olives. Seal and relax for a maximum of 4 days.

Reheat in the microwave for about 2 minutes until heated through, to serve. Just before eating dress up with tahini sauce.

> Daily total nutritional analysis: 1,213 calories, 59 grams protein, 31 grams fiber, 143 grams carbohydrates, 2,134 mg sodium, 51 grams fat.

## DAY NINETEEN

**Breakfast: Pineapple Green Smoothie** (297 calories) - Check above for recipe

**Morning Snack:** 2 plums (61 calories)

**Lunch: Instant Pot White Chicken Chilli Freezer Pack** with a side of 2 celery stalks and 3 tablespoons of hummus (346 calories) - Check Above for Recipe

**Evening Snack:** ¾ cup blueberries (63 calories)

**Dinner: Vegetarian Spaghetti Squash Lasagna with** a side dish of 2 cups mixed greens topped with 1 tablespoon of **Basil Vinaigrette** (416 calories)

**Ingredients**

- 1½ to 3 pound spaghetti squash, halved lengthwise and seeded
- ¼ cup water
- 2 tablespoons extra virgin olive oil
- 1 medium onion, chopped
- 4 cloves garlic, minced
- 10 oz. mushrooms, sliced
- 2 cups crushed tomatoes
- 1 teaspoon Italian seasoning
- ½ teaspoon ground pepper, divided
- ¼ teaspoon crushed red pepper
- ¼ teaspoon salt, divided
- ¼ cup grated Parmesan cheese
- 1 cup shredded part-skim mozzarella cheese, divided
- ½ cup part-skim ricotta cheese

## How to Prepare

1. In the upper third of the oven, place rack; preheat to 450°F (230°C).

2. In a microwave-safe bowl, put squash cut-side down, and add water. Microwave, uncovered, 10-12 minutes on high until the flesh is soft. (Alternatively, put the squash cut-side down on a large rimmed baking sheet. Bake at 400°F (200°C) until tender, 40 to 50 minutes.)

3. In the meantime, heat oil over medium heat in a large skillet. Add onion and garlic; cook, stirring, for 3-4 minutes until beginning to soften.

4. Add mushrooms and cook for about 5 minutes, stirring, until the vegetables are tender and begin to brown. Add tomatoes, seasoning with Italian, ¼ teaspoon pepper, crushed red pepper and ⅛ teaspoon salt. Cook for 1-2 minutes until heated and flavors have mixed. Switch off heat and cover.

5. Use a fork to scrape the squash from the shells the into a large bowl. Stir the remaining ¼ teaspoon pepper and ⅛ teaspoon salt in Parmesan. Drop the cut-side up shells onto a wide rimmed baking sheet. Squash-Parmesan spoon ¼ of the mixture into each container. Tomato mixture layer ¼ on top, then scatter ¼ cup mozzarella into each shell. Dollop ricotta with ¼ cup over the mozzarella. Repeat with remaining mixture of onion, tomato sauce, and mozzarella.

6. Bake lasagnas with squash for 15 minutes. Switch the broiler to high and broil, watch closely, 1-2 minutes, until the cheese begins to brown. For serving, break each lasagna in half.

Daily total nutritional analysis: 1,183 calories, 38 grams fiber, 62 grams protein, 170 grams carbohydrates, 37 grams fat, 1,901 mg sodium.

## DAY TWENTY

**Breakfast: Creamy Blueberry-Pecan Overnight Oatmeal** (291 calories) - Check above for Recipe

**Morning Snack:** ¾ cup raspberries (48 calories)

**Lunch: Mediterranean Tuna-Spinach Salad** (375 calories) - Check above for Recipe

**Evening Snack:** ¾ cup blackberries (46 calories)

**Dinner: Hasselback Caprese Chicken** with 1½ cups **Roasted Fresh Green Beans** (443 calories)

**Ingredients**

- 2 boneless, skinless chicken breasts (8 oz. each)
- ½ teaspoon salt, divided
- ½ teaspoon ground pepper, divided
- 1 medium tomato, sliced
- 3 oz. fresh mozzarella, halved and sliced

- ¼ cup prepared pesto
- 8 cups broccoli florets
- 2 tablespoons extra virgin olive oil

## How to Prepare

1. Preheat oven to 375°F (190°C). Coat with the cooking spray on a wide rimmed baking sheet.

2. Allow through ½ inch crosswise cuts along both chicken breasts, slicing almost to the bottom but not all the way through. Sprinkle with ¼ teaspoon of chicken each with salt and pepper. Alternately fill in the cuts with slices of tomato and mozzarella. Cover with pesto. Move the chicken onto one side of the baking sheet prepared.

3. In a large bowl, toss broccoli, oil and the remaining ¼ teaspoon with every salt and pepper. If any slices of tomatoes are left, mix them in. Place the broccoli mixture onto the empty side of the baking sheet.

4. Bake until the chicken in the center is no longer pink, and the broccoli is tender, about 25 minutes. Halve each breast and serve with broccoli

Daily total nutritional analysis: 1,203 calories, 116 grams carbohydrates, 34 grams fiber, 77 g protein,1,458 mg sodium, 55 grams fat.

## DAY TWENTY-ONE

**Breakfast: Pineapple Green Smoothie** (297 calories) - Check above for Recipe

**Morning snack:** 2 plums (61 calories)

**Lunch: Mediterranean Tuna-Spinach Salad** (375 calories) - Check above for Recipe

**Evening Snack:** 1 cup sliced cucumbers, squeeze of lemon juice, salt and pepper to taste (16 calories)

**Dinner: Stuffed Sweet Potato with Hummus Dressing** (472 calories)

## Ingredients

- 1 large sweet potato, scrubbed
- ¾ cup chopped kale
- 1 cup canned black beans, rinsed
- ¼ cup hummus
- 2 tablespoons water

## How to Prepare

1. Prick sweet potato with a fork all over. Microwave on high for 7-10 minutes, until cooked through.

2. Meanwhile, wash the kale and drain. Layer in a medium sauce-pan; cover over medium-high heat and cook until wilted, stirring once or twice. Add beans; if the ingredients begin sticking to the pot, add a spoonful or two of water. Continue to cook, uncovered, stir occasionally, for 1-2 minutes, until the mixture is steaming.

3. Break open the sweet potato and cover with mixture of kale and beans. Combine the hummus in a small dish with 2 table-spoons of water to create a dressing. Add extra water to achieve desired consistency as needed. Drizzle the hummus dressing over the stuffed sweet potato.

---

Daily total nutritional analysis: 1,221 calories, 61 grams protein, 184 grams carbohydrates, 40 grams fiber, 34 grams fat, 1,587 mg sodium.

---

## DAY TWENTY-TWO

**Breakfast: Pineapple Green Smoothie** (297 calories) - Check above for Recipe

**Morning Snack:** 1 cup blackberries (62 calories)

**Lunch:** 1 **salmon fillet (remainder from Sweet & Spicy Roasted Salmon Plus Wild Rice Pilaf)** also 1 cup **Roasted Butternut Squash & Root Vegetables** and ⅓ cup **Lemon-Roasted Mixed Vegetables** (354 calories)

**Evening Snack:** 1 large peach (68 calories)

**Dinner: Green Salad with Edamame & Beets** topped with ¼ of an avocado (405 calories)

**Ingredients**

- 2 cups mixed salad greens
- 1 cup shelled edamame, thawed
- ½ medium raw beet, peeled and shredded (about ½ cup)
- 1 tablespoon plus 1½ teaspoons red-wine vinegar
- 1 tablespoon chopped fresh cilantro
- 2 teaspoons extra virgin olive oil
- Freshly ground pepper to taste

**How to Prepare**

Arrange greens, edamame and beet on a large plate. Whisk vinegar, cilantro, oil, salt and pepper in a small bowl. Drizzle over the salad and enjoy.

Daily total nutritional analysis: 1,187 calories,151 grams carbohydrates, 44 grams fiber, 42 grams fat, 1,354 mg sodium,63 grams protein.

# DAY TWENTY-THREE

**Breakfast: Muesli with Raspberries** (287 calories) - Check above for recipe

**Morning Snack:** 1 plum (30 calories)

**Lunch: Piled-High Greek Vegetable Pitas** (399 calories)

**Ingredients**

- 1 tablespoon olive oil
- 1 cup canned no-salt-added chickpeas (garbanzo beans), rinsed and patted dry
- ½ teaspoon paprika
- ¼ teaspoon garlic powder
- ¼ teaspoon ground cumin
- ⅛ teaspoon ground pepper
- 2 cups Roasted Butternut Squash & Root Vegetables (see Associated Recipes)
- 1⅓ cups Lemon-Roasted Mixed Vegetables (see Associated Recipes)
- 1 cup fresh baby spinach
- ½ cup cherry tomatoes, halved
- ¼ cup crumbled reduced-fat feta cheese (1 oz.)
- 2 (6-7 inch) whole-wheat pita bread rounds, halved horizontally and lightly toasted
- ½ cup hummus
- Lemon wedges

**How to Prepare**

1. Steam oil over medium heat, in a 10 inch skillet. Remove the chickpeas, sprinkle with paprika, ground garlic, cumin and pepper. Cook, stirring frequently, for 6-8 minutes, until the chickpeas are lightly browned.

2. The chickpeas are moved to a medium bowl. Add roasted butternut squash & root vegetables, lemon-roasted mixed vegetables, spinach, tomatoes, and feta; gently mix together. Serve with wedges of pita, hummus, and lime.

**Evening Snack:** 1 cup sliced red bell pepper (29 calories)

**Dinner: Slow-Cooker Pasta e Fagioli Soup Freezer Pack** (457 calories) - Check above for Recipe

Daily Total nutritional analysis: 1,202 calories, 63 grams protein, 160 g carbohydrates, 36 grams fiber, 40 grams fat, 1,461 mg sodium.

## DAY TWENTY-FOUR

**Breakfast: Everything Bagel Avocado Toast** with a side of 1 hard-boiled egg (250 calories) - Check above for Recipe

**Morning Snack:** ⅔ cup raspberries (42 calories)

**Lunch: Piled-High Greek Vegetable Pitas** (399 calories) - Check above for Recipe

**Evening Snack:** 1 plum (30 calories)

**Dinner: Quinoa, Chicken and Broccoli Salad** plus **Roasted Lemon Dressing** (481 calories)

**Ingredients**

- 1 (8 oz.) boneless, skinless chicken breast, trimmed
- 4 tablespoons extra virgin olive oil, divided
- ⅛ teaspoon salt plus ¼ teaspoon, divided
- 2 small lemons, thinly sliced and seeded
- 1 cup low-sodium chicken broth
- ½ cup quinoa
- 8 oz. broccoli with stems (about 1 medium head)
- ¼ cup red-wine vinegar

- 1 tablespoon Dijon mustard
- 2 cups arugula
- ¾ cup chopped walnuts, toasted
- ½ cup dried cranberries
- ½ cup chopped fresh mint

## How to Prepare

1. Preheat oven to 425°F (220°C).

2. Layer the chicken in a rimmed baking sheet on one side. Attach 1 spoonful of oil and sprinkle with ⅛ teaspoon salt. Fry for ten minutes. Layer lemon slices across from the baking sheet. Roast, turn once, until an instant-read thermometer inserted into the chicken's thickest part hits 160°F (70°C) and the lemons are browned (typically another 7-9 minutes).

3. Meanwhile in a small saucepan, add broth and quinoa to a boil. Reduce heat to keep the liquid boiling, cover and cook for about 15 minutes, until the liquid is absorbed. Remove from heat, and let stand for 10 minutes, covered.

4. Cut off stems of broccoli florets. Cut, peel, and dice the stems thinly, and cut the florets into bits of bite size.

5. Chop half the slices of lemon. Combine the remaining 3 table-spoons of oil and ¼ teaspoon salt in a large bowl with the vinegar, mustard and mustard.

6. Shred the chicken. Apply to dressing the chicken, the remaining slices of lemon, broccoli, quinoa, arugula, walnuts, cranberries and mint; shake to mix.

Daily Total nutritional analysis: 1,202 calories, 50 grams protein, 33 grams fiber, 1,403 mg sodium 131 grams carbohydrates, 57 grams fat

# DAY TWENTY-FIVE

**Breakfast: Blueberry Almond Chia Pudding** (229 calories)

## Ingredients

- ½ cup unsweetened almond milk or other non-dairy milk beverage
- 2 tablespoons chia seeds
- 2 teaspoons pure maple syrup
- ⅛ teaspoon almond extract
- ½ cup fresh blueberries, divided
- 1 tablespoon toasted slivered almonds, divided

**How to Prepare**

1. In a small bowl, mix almond milk (or any other non-dairy milk beverage), chia, maple syrup and almond extract. Cover and refrigerate for a total of 8 hours, up to 3 days.

2. When the pudding is ready to serve, mix well. In a serving glass (or bowl), spoon around half of the pudding and top with half of the blueberries and almonds. Add the rest of the pudding and finish with remaining almonds and blueberries.

**Morning Snack:** 5 oz. non-fat plain Greek yogurt plus ¼ cup blueberries and 1 tablespoon of chopped walnuts (153 calories)

**Lunch: Piled-High Greek Vegetable Pitas** (399 calories) - Check above for Recipe

**Evening Snack:** 1 big peach (68 calories)

**Dinner: Mediterranean Cod with Roasted Tomatoes and ¾ cup Quinoa Avocado Salad** (364 calories)

Daily total nutritional analysis: 1,213 calories, 140 grams carbohydrates, 49 grams fat 65 grams protein, 140 grams carbohydrates, 35 grams fiber 1,450 mg sodium.

## DAY TWENTY-SIX

**Breakfast: Everything Bagel Avocado Toast** with a side dish of one hard-boiled egg (250 calories) - Check above for Recipe

**Morning Snack:** 1 cup raspberries (64 calories)

**Lunch: Piled-High Greek Vegetable Pitas** (399 calories) - Check above for Recipe

**Evening Snack:** 5 oz. non-fat plain Greek yogurt plus ⅓ cup blackberries (104 calories)

**Dinner: Caprese Stuffed Portobello Mushrooms** with ¾ cup Quinoa Avocado Salad (393 calories)

**Ingredients**

- 3 tablespoons extra virgin olive oil, divided
- 1 medium clove garlic, minced
- ½ teaspoon salt, divided
- ½ teaspoon ground pepper, divided
- 4 portobello mushrooms (about 14 oz.), stems and gills removed (see Tip)
- 1 cup halved cherry tomatoes
- ½ cup fresh mozzarella pearls, drained and patted dry
- ½ cup thinly sliced fresh basil
- 2 teaspoons best-quality balsamic vinegar

**How to Prepare**

1. Preheat oven to 400°F (200°C).

2. In a small bowl, mix 2 tablespoons of butter, garlic, ¼ teaspoon salt and ¼ teaspoon pepper. Coat mushrooms all over with the oil mixture, using a silicone brush. Place on a wide rimmed baking sheet and bake for about 10 minutes, until the mushrooms are mostly tender.

3. Meanwhile, in a medium bowl, whisk together tomatoes, mozzarella, basil and the remaining ¼ teaspoon salt, ¼ teaspoon pepper and 1 tablespoon oil. Extract from the oven once the mushrooms have cooled, and cover with tomato mixture. Bake until the cheese is completely melted, and the tomatoes wilted, around 12-15 minutes longer. Add ½ teaspoon vinegar to each mushroom, and drink.

---

Daily total nutritional analysis: 1,210 calories, 124 grams carbohydrates, 60 grams fat, 54 grams protein, 37 grams fiber, 1,559 mg sodium.

---

## DAY TWENTY-SEVEN

**Breakfast: Muesli with Raspberries** (287 calories) - Check above for Recipe

**Morning Snack:** 1 large peach (68 calories)

**Lunch: Instant Pot White Chicken Chilli Freezer Pack plus ½ cup blueberries** (298 calories) - Check above for Recipe

**Evening Snack:** ¾ cup sliced red bell pepper with 1 tablespoon hummus (47 calories)

**Dinner: Stuffed Eggplant with 1 serving Traditional Greek Salad** (513 calories)

Daily Totals: 1,214 calories, 157 g carbohydrates, 54 grams protein, 39 grams fiber, 49 grams fat, 1,739 mg sodium.

## DAY TWENTY-EIGHT

**Breakfast: Berry-Mint Kefir Smoothies** (274 calories) - Check above for Recipe

**Morning Snack:** ½ cup sliced red bell pepper (14 calories)

**Lunch: Instant Pot White Chicken Chilli Freezer Pack** with ½ cup blueberries (298 calories) - Check above for Recipe

**Evening Snack:** ½ cup sliced cucumbers with a pinch of salt & pepper (8 calories)

**Dinner: Chickpea Pasta with Lemony-Parsley Pesto** (630 calories)

**Ingredients**

- 4 oz. chickpea penne or other penne pasta (about 1¼ cups dry)
- 1 bunch flat-leaf parsley (about 4 cups lightly packed), plus more for garnish
- 3 cloves garlic
- ⅓ cup extra virgin olive oil
- 1 teaspoon lemon zest
- 2 tablespoons lemon juice
- ½ teaspoon kosher salt
- ¼ teaspoon ground black pepper

- 1½ cups roasted root vegetables

**How to Prepare**

1. Cook pasta according to the instructions on the box and drain once cooked.

2. At the same time, in a food processor, combine the parsley and garlic and pulse until chopped evenly, about 10 times. Apply butter, lemon juice, salt and pepper, and puree for about 15 seconds until just combined; it should be chunky.

3. Microwave roasted root vegetables in a microwave-safe bowl for about 1 minute, until heated through. (Alternatively, heat 1 teaspoon of extra virgin olive oil over medium - high heat in a large skillet. Add vegetables and cook, stirring frequently, until warm, for 2-4 minutes.) Throw the hot pasta with the pesto, vegetables and lemon zest. If needed, garnish with parsley.

Daily total nutritional analysis: 1,224 calories, 53 g protein, 154 g carbohydrates, 33 g fiber, 50 g fat, 1,491 mg sodium.

# CHAPTER 8
# BREAKFAST AND STARTERS RECIPES

## 1. Mediterranean Breakfast Tostadas

Preparation Time: 15 minutes

Serving: 4 servings

**Ingredients**

- 8 eggs (beaten)
- ½ cup skimmed milk
- 4 tostadas
- ½ cup red pepper (diced)
- ¼ cup feta crumbled
- ½ cup green onions (chopped)
- ½ cup roasted red pepper hummus
- ½ teaspoon oregano
- ½ cup tomatoes diced
- ½ teaspoon garlic powder

**How to Prepare**

1. Cook the red peppers for about two to three minutes in a large non-stick pot over medium heat, until it becomes tender.

2. Add the oregano, milk, egg, garlic powder and green onions to the bowl, while stirring continuously until the egg whites are no more translucent (this will take about 2 minutes).

3. Add mixture of eggs, tomatoes, hummus, cucumber, and feta on each tostada. Serve the food straight away.

## 2. Oatmeal with Raisins, Nuts and Apple

Preparation time: 7 hours 10 minutes

Serving: 6 servings

**Ingredients**

- 3 ½ cups fat-free milk
- ½ teaspoon salt
- 1 large apple, peeled and chopped
- 4 ½ teaspoons butter, melted
- ¾ cup steel-cut oats
- ¾ cup raisins
- 3 tablespoons brown sugar
- ¾ teaspoon ground cinnamon
- ¼ cup chopped pecan

**How to Prepare**

1. In a slow cooker that was sprayed with cooking spray earlier, mix all the ingredients except the chopped pecans.

2. Cover the mixture and cook on low for about 7 to 8 hours or until you note that the mixture has been absorbed. Serve the oatmeal into bowls and garnish with pecans afterwards.

This recipe is perfect when you want to wake up with the breakfast waiting for you. Just measure out your ingredients right before bed and turn your slow cooker on to LOW and let it cook overnight.

## 3. Fig and Honey Yogurt

Preparation Time 5 minutes

Serving: 1 serving

## Ingredients

- ⅔ cup low-fat plain yogurt
- 2 teaspoons honey
- 3 dried figs (sliced)

## How to Prepare

1. Put the yogurt in a bowl and top it with figs and honey

## 4. Vegetable Frittata

Preparation Time: 30 minutes

Serving: 4 servings

## Ingredients

- ⅓ cup milk
- ½ teaspoon salt
- 8 large eggs
- 2 teaspoon olive oil
- ¼ teaspoon pepper
- 1 medium sized red bell pepper, seeded and thinly sliced
- ½ small sized red onion, thinly sliced (this is about ½ cup)
- 2 cups packed baby spinach
- 4 oz. feta

## How to Prepare

1. With the rack in the center, preheat your oven to 350°F (180°C). Whisk the eggs in a large container of milk, salt, and pepper.

2. Heat oil over moderate heat in a 10 inch oven-safe dish. Add onion and red pepper to it and sauté until softened for about 7 minutes.

3. Stir in spinach and sauté for about 2 minutes, until wilted. Spread vegetables evenly in skillet and pour in the mixture of the eggs. Crumble feta over mixture.

4. Cook without stirring until eggs are just beginning to set around the edges, 2-3 minutes.

5. Place skillet in oven. Bake frittata until almost set in centre, about 15 minutes. Turn broiler on high. Broil frittata until the top is golden brown, about 2 minutes, watching carefully to prevent over-browning. Remove from oven. Let frittata rest for 5 minutes before serving.

## 5. Avo-Tahini Toast

Preparation time: 5 minutes

Serving: 1 serving

**Ingredients**

- 1 teaspoon fresh lemon juice
- Dash of kosher salt
- slice whole-grain bread, toasted
- 1 teaspoon tahini (sesame paste)
- 3 grape tomatoes, quartered
- ½ ripe peeled avocado 1 (1-ounce)
- 2 pitted kalamata olives, chopped
- 1 hard-cooked large egg, peeled and sliced

**How to Prepare**

1. In a bowl, combine the juice, salt, and avocado, mashing with a fork.

2. Spread avocado mixture evenly over toast; top with tomatoes, olives, and egg. Drizzle with tahini.

## 6. Cheesy Apple Raisin Cinnamon Omelet

Serving: 4 servings

## Ingredients

- 1 medium sweet apple (Fiji, Fuji, or Golden Delicious), peeled, cored, and sliced
- 1 tablespoon extra virgin olive oil
- 2 tablespoons seedless black raisins
- 1 cup egg substitute or 1 cup egg whites or 4 whole eggs
- 2 tablespoons crumbled blue cheese
- 2 tablespoons freshly shredded Parmesan cheese
- Salt and freshly ground pepper to taste
- ⅛ teaspoon cinnamon

## How to Prepare

1. Fry the slices of apples in ½ tablespoon of olive oil until crispy

2. Add in raisins, then immediately remove the apple mix from the casserole, and transfer to a dish.

3. Combine the bacon, cheeses, salt and pepper and blend well.

4. Melt remaining olive oil into omelette pan 5. Cook ¼ of the mixture of eggs at a time, raising the edges at low heat to allow the uncooked portion to flow and cook under.

6. Repeat the process for each serving 4 times.

7. Arrange ¼ of the mixture of apples over half the cooked egg.

8. Fold in half, and sprinkle over with cinnamon.


# 7. Poached Eggs in a Garden

Serving: 4 servings

## Ingredients

- 2 tablespoons olive oil
- 2 large russet potatoes (diced)

- 2 cups fresh broccoli florets
- 1 medium red bell pepper (chopped)
- 1 medium white onion (chopped)
- 2 cups button mushrooms (sliced)
- Salt and freshly ground pepper (to taste)
- 8 large eggs (poached)

## How to Prepare

1. Heat the olive oil over medium-high heat in a large skillet.

2. To your taste, add potatoes, broccoli, red bell pepper, cabbage, mushrooms, salt and pepper.

3. Cook until vegetables are tender, and potatoes begin to turn brown, stirring occasionally.

4. Divide into 4 servings and serve with 2 poached eggs on top of each serving.

# 8. Spanish Omelette

Serving: 6 main course servings

## Ingredients

- 2 tablespoons extra virgin olive oil
- 6 whole scallions (coarsely chopped)
- 4 cloves fresh garlic (thinly sliced)
- 1 green bell pepper (seeded and thinly sliced)
- 1 red bell pepper (seeded and thinly sliced)
- 1 medium zucchini (diced)
- 3 ripe tomatoes (peeled and cut into wedges)
- Salt and freshly ground pepper to taste
- ¼ teaspoon cayenne pepper
- ¾ teaspoon ground cumin
- ½ teaspoon ground coriander

- ½ teaspoon ground cinnamon
- 4 tablespoons chopped fresh parsley
- 3 cups egg substitute or 3 cups egg whites or 12 large eggs
- ¼ pound crumbled fresh low-fat goat's cheese

## How to Prepare

1. Heat 2 tablespoons of olive oil and sauté scallions and garlic gently for about 5 minutes in an oven-safe skillet, until they start softening.

2. Add the green and red bell peppers, zucchini, and tomatoes, heat up slightly and continue sautéing for another five to ten minutes until the vegetables have softened and most of the juice has been absorbed.

3. Cover with pepper and salt and set aside at room temperature.

4. Combine the herbs and the eggs in a large bowl and mix just enough to break the yolks with a fork.

5. Use a slotted spoon to extract the vegetables from the skillet and combine them with eggs. Put the skillet back on the medium heat, then add more olive oil if necessary.

6. Add the eggs and vegetable mixture when the olive oil is hot, and cook for about 2 to 3 minutes, raising the edges under the cooked ones with a spatula to allow uncooked eggs to run under.

7. Crumble the goat's cheese over the top of the omelet and shift the skillet to a 400°F (200°C) oven to finish cooking for around 15 to 20 minutes, or until the omelet is already and the cheese is melted.

## 9. Vegetable Omelette with Pesto

Serving: 6 servings

**Ingredients**

- ½ teaspoon extra virgin olive oil
- 1 cup sliced white mushrooms
- ⅔ medium red onion (diced)
- ½ cup fresh peas, cooked and drained 2 whole carrots, cleaned, cut julienne style, cooked, and drained (you can substitute with other vegetables, if desired)
- 2 tablespoons Basil Pesto Sauce or a market-fresh pesto sauce
- Olive oil cooking spray
- 3 cups egg substitute or 3 cups egg whites or 12 whole fresh eggs
- ¼ cup water
- ¼ teaspoon salt
- ¼ teaspoon freshly ground pepper
- 6 sprigs fresh basil for garnish

**How to Prepare**

1. Heat the olive oil and sauté the mushrooms and onion in a medium skillet, then remove from heat.

2. Add all other mushroom and onion vegetables and add in prepared pesto. Sprinkle with olive oil spray a non-stick baking pan and set aside.

3. Combine the eggs with water and salt and pepper in a mixing bowl. Beat until foamy. Pour the egg mixture in the pan and bake uncovered for about 8 minutes at 400°F (200°C), or until mixture is set. Cut baked eggs into about 5 inch squares and cut squares from pot.

4. On half of each omelet square, spoon ¼ cup vegetable mixture, fold over and garnish with basil sprigs.

## 10.    Broccoli and Cheese Frittata

Servin: 6 main course servings

## Ingredients

- 3 cups broccoli florets
- 1 tablespoon extra virgin olive oil
- ½ cup finely chopped onion
- ½ cup chopped red bell pepper
- 2 cloves fresh garlic (minced)
- 1 cup shredded mozzarella cheese
- A dash of crushed red-hot pepper flakes
- 1½ cups egg substitute or 1½ cups egg whites or 6 large eggs
- Olive oil spray

## How to Prepare

1. Steam broccoli until soft, crispy and remove from heat. Heat olive oil and sauté onion, bell pepper, and garlic in a large skillet over medium-high heat until the vegetables are soft (about 5 minutes).

2. Remove broccoli and cook for about 2 minutes. Transfer the vegetable mixture to a bowl, then add hot pepper flakes and mozzarella cheese. If using whole eggs, beat until blended in a separate bowl.

3. Transfer the eggs into a vegetable mixture and pour them into a round cake pan that is lightly sprayed with olive oil. Bake in a 325°F (160°C) oven for about 30 minutes, until the eggs are set. Serve them warm or at room temperature.

## 11.    Ham and Zucchini Frittata

Serving: 6 servings

## Ingredients

- 1 tablespoon olive oil
- 1 medium white onion (chopped)

- 1 clove fresh garlic (minced)
- 1 medium zucchini, halved lengthwise cut to ¼ inch thick slices
- 1 cup diced low-sodium ham
- 1½ cups liquid eggs
- ¼ cup low-fat milk
- 1 teaspoon dry Italian seasoning mix plus more to sprinkle
- Salt and freshly ground pepper to taste
- 2 Italian plum tomatoes (sliced)
- 1 cup shredded, part-skim milk mozzarella cheese

**How to Prepare**

1. Preheat oven to 325°F (160°C). Heat the olive oil inside an oven-safe skillet over medium heat. Add the onion, garlic and zucchini, then sauté until smooth. Reduce the heat to low-medium, add ham and cook for 2 minutes.

2. Combine liquid eggs, milk, Italian seasoning mixture and salt and pepper into a bowl to taste.

3. Pour mixture with ham into the skillet and cook unstirred for about five minutes or until the eggs start to set.

4. Arrange the tomato slices and scatter with mozzarella cheese on top of the egg mixture. Place skillet about 6 inches under broiler and broil for about four to five minutes until the eggs are ready and cheese is lightly browned.

5. Sprinkle with a splash of Italian seasoning mix and serve over the frittata.

## 12.    Quinoa and Raisins Porridge

Serving: 2 large servings

**Ingredients**

- 2 cups almond milk
- 1 cup quinoa that has been rinsed through a fine mesh sieve under cold water
- ½ teaspoon ground cinnamon
- ⅛ teaspoon ground nutmeg
- ⅛ teaspoon ground ginger
- Dash of salt (optional)
- 2 tablespoons pure maple syrup
- ½ teaspoon pure vanilla extract
- 2 tablespoons raisins
- ¼ cup chopped nuts (such as pecans, walnuts, or almonds)

**How to Prepare**

1. Gently heat the almond milk in a saucepan over medium heat, stirring occasionally until it begins to bubble. Simmer heat and add quinoa, cinnamon, nutmeg, ginger and butter. Cook uncovered until quinoa is tender and starts to thicken (about 20–25 minutes) while stirring occasionally.

2. Remove from heat and add the vanilla extract, maple syrup, and raisins. Put a sprinkling of nuts over it and serve.

## 13.    Mixed Vegetable Frittata

Serving:4 servings

**Ingredients**

- 10 large fresh asparagus spears
- 1½ cups egg substitute or 1½ cups egg whites or 6 whole eggs
- ¾ cup low-fat cottage cheese
- 2 teaspoons spicy brown mustard
- ¼ teaspoon crushed dried tarragon
- ¼ teaspoon marjoram
- Salt and freshly ground pepper to taste

- ½ teaspoon extra virgin olive oil
- 1 cup sliced fresh mushrooms
- ½ cup diced onion
- ¼ cup chopped seeded tomato for garnish

## How to Prepare

1. Boil asparagus for eight to ten minutes until tender and crispy. Drain it. Cut the spears into 1 inch pieces, except 3. Hold it on top. Mix the bacon, cottage cheese, mustard, tarragon, marjoram, salt and pepper in a bowl to taste. Put it aside.

2. In a large oven-safe skillet, heat olive oil, and sauté the mushrooms and onion until tender. Stir in pieces of asparagus, add egg mixture over top and cook another 5 minutes at low heat until it bubbles and starts to set.

3. Arrange 3 uncut asparagus spears that sit on top of the mixture. Put the skillet inside the oven and bake for 10 minutes at 400°F (200°C) uncovered, or until the frittata sets. Take out of the oven and garnish with tomato.

## 14. Zucchini Frittata

Serving: 6 servings

## Ingredients

- 1½ tablespoons extra virgin olive oil
- 1 medium yellow onion, chopped
- 2 cloves fresh garlic, minced
- 3 small zucchini, sliced ¼-ich thick
- Salt and freshly ground pepper to taste
- 2 tablespoons minced fresh basil leaves
- 2 cups egg substitute or 2 cups egg whites or 8 large eggs
- ½ cup (2 oz.) freshly grated Parmesan cheese

## How to Prepare

1. In a skillet, heat olive oil over low-medium heat and sauté onion and garlic until soft and light brown. Add the zucchini and salt and pepper to the garlic onion mixture and cook for another 5 to 8 minutes.

2. Take off heat and set aside. In a bowl, add basil and eggs to the zucchini mixture (beat eggs, if using whole eggs).

3. Stir the mixture into a lightly greased round cake pan to blend and add the egg mixture in. Bake 325°F (160°C) in an oven, until the eggs are set.

4. Sprinkle Parmesan cheese over frittata, remove from the oven and put under broiler for 2–3 minutes until the cheese is golden brown. Remove from the oven and eat immediately.

## 15. Tunisian Egg, Tuna, and Tomato Sandwiches

Serving: 4 servings

**Ingredients**

- ¼ cup (60 ml) extra virgin olive oil
- 2 cloves garlic (minced)
- ½ small yellow onion (minced)
- ½ small green bell pepper (stemmed seeded, and minced)
- 1 medium ripe tomato (diced)
- Unrefined sea salt or salt, to taste
- Freshly ground black pepper, to taste
- 4 small hero or sandwich rolls
- 1 small English cucumber (thinly sliced)
- 1 medium ripe tomato (thinly sliced)
- 9 or 10 oz. which is about (255 to 283 g) tuna in olive oil (well drained)
- 2 hardboiled eggs, (sliced into quarters)

- ½ cup (or 50 g) pitted black olives
- 4 jarred pepperoncini peppers, (drained, stemmed, and halved in length)
- ½ cup (or 120 g) harissa or any other hot sauce

**How to Prepare**

1. Heat up the olive oil over medium-high heat in a large skillet. Add the garlic, onion, pepper, and diced tomato and cook until soft, about 6 minutes, through continuous stirring.

2. Season with salt and chilli pepper and set aside. Split the rolls horizontally, to one leg, leaving them intact. Divide the tomato sauce into wraps, cover with cucumber, sliced tomato and then tuna 3. Finish it with the olives, cheese, and pepperoncini. Drizzle with harissa and serve on top of each.

## 16.    Seasonal Italian Frittata

Serving: 4 servings

**Ingredients**

- ¼ cup (or 60 ml) of extra virgin olive oil
- ½ medium yellow onion, (cut into very thin slices)
- 1 pint (or 175 g) shitake mushrooms, (stemmed and cut into very thin slices ⅛ inch or 3 mm slices)
- 2 small leeks or 1 large leek (light green and white parts rinsed and finely chopped)
- 8 basil leaves which have been hand torn
- 6 large eggs, beaten in a bowl until frothy
- ¼ cup (30 g) of grated Pecorino Romano
- 1 teaspoon unrefined sea salt or salt

**How to Prepare**

1. Heat the oven beforehand to 350°F (180°C). Heat up the oil over medium-high heat in a big, wide, ovenproof skillet.

2. Add the onion with sauté and stirring occasionally until soft and translucent, about 4 minutes in colour. Stir in the mushrooms and brown for 4 minutes. Attach the leeks, stir and continue cooking for another 4 minutes.

3. Remove the basil leaves, beat chickens, roman pecorino, and salt. Mix well, and you reduce to medium-low heat. Cook for about 4 to 5 minutes, without stirring, or until the eggs are cooked through and through.

4. To finish the frittata cooking, place the skillet in the oven until the top of the frittata is golden and the eggs are set. Cut into 4 pieces, then serve.

## 17.    Israeli Shakshouka–Style Eggs

Serving: 4 servings

### Ingredients

- 2 tablespoons (30 ml) extra virgin olive oil
- 2 tablespoons (30 g) harissa sauce or hot sauce
- 2 tablespoons (32 g) tomato paste
- 1 teaspoon smoked paprika
- 1 yellow onion (diced)
- 2 large red peppers (trimmed, seeded, and cut into small pieces)
- 3 cups (or 678 g) chopped very ripe tomatoes
- 6 large organic eggs
- ½ cup (115 g) Labneh or otherwise plain Greek yogurt
- 4 pieces Whole-Wheat Pita Bread or another pita (warmed, for serving)

### How to Prepare

1. Heat the olive oil over moderate heat in a large skillet, then add the harissa, tomato paste, paprika, onion and peppers. Combine

well and allow to cook until the peppers are tender which is about 5-7 minutes.

2. Add the tomatoes, stir and raise to high heat. When the mixture starts to boil, reduce heat to low and simmer for about 10 minutes until the sauce is thickened. Taste the seasoning and adjust if necessary.

3. Build 6 wells into the sauce. Into the wells crack eggs. The egg whites gently float into the sauce using a fork. Simmer, uncovered, till the whites of the eggs are set but the yolks of the eggs are not yet firm, about 6 to 8 minutes.

4. Remove from heat and allow to set before serving for a few minutes. Serve with yogurt or labneh, and soft pita bread.

## 18.    Omelette Provencale

Serving: 4 servings

### Ingredients

- 2 tablespoons (30 ml) extra virgin olive oil, plus extra 2 teaspoons for serving
- 2 zucchini (diced)
- 2 roasted red peppers from a jar (drained and finely chopped)
- 1 clove garlic, finely chopped
- ¼ cup (12 g) finely chopped chives
- 8 eggs
- ½ teaspoon unrefined sea salt or salt
- ¼ teaspoon freshly ground black pepper
- 2½ oz. (½ cup, or 38 g) goat cheese
- 2 tablespoons (5 g) finely chopped fresh basil
- 4 cups (100 g), mixed field greens, baby spinach, or arugula, to serve
- 1 teaspoon lemon juice

## How to Prepare

1. In a large skillet, heat 2 tablespoons (30 ml) of olive oil over medium heat. Afterwards, add the zucchini, roasted red pepper, garlic, and chives, then cook gently until softened for about 10 minutes.

2. Break the eggs into a cup, whisk gently, and add salt and pepper to season. Pour the eggs into the pan, turn them around and swivel to the suit. Add the goat's cheese knobs over the top then sprinkle with basil.

3. Cook until the egg is set and browned lightly underneath, then cover the pan with a plate and invert the omelette onto it. Slide it back into the other side of the pan to cook.

4. Divide 1 cup or 25 g of salad greens on 4 plates and chop with remaining olive oil and lemon juice to serve. Serve the omelette folded around the fillings.

# CHAPTER 9
# APPETIZERS RECIPES

## 19.    Roasted Garlic

Serving: 4 to 5 servings

**Ingredients**

- 1 jumbo fresh elephant garlic head
- Extra virgin olive oil to drizzle
- Dry seasonings of choice (optional)

**How to Prepare**

1. Holding entire head of garlic, cut off the top leaf points of each clove to expose a small portion of the clove.

2. Keep the remainder of leaves intact around the body of the garlic head. Place trimmed garlic head in a tight-fitting oven-safe bowl, trimmed side up.

3. Drizzle a little olive oil over the top of the head and down around the sides. Sprinkle with your favorite seasoning(optional).

4. Place garlic on middle rack of oven and bake at 400°F (200°C) for 20 to 30 minutes or until cloves are soft and a light golden brown.

5. Remove from oven and spread garlic on crusty bread or add to vegetables, omelets, or pasta.

# 20. Stuffed Grape Leaves (Dolmas)

Serving: 20 servings

## Ingredients

- 3 tablespoon an extra virgin olive oil, divided
- 1 cup chopped red onion
- ½ cup chopped scallions
- 1 cup basmati rice
- 4 cloves fresh garlic, minced
- 1 teaspoon ground cumin
- ½ teaspoon freshly ground pepper
- 2 cups canned low-sodium vegetable broth
- ¼ cup chopped fennel
- ¼ cup chopped fresh dill
- ¼ cup finely chopped fresh parsley
- 2 tablespoons dried mint
- 1 (16 oz.) jar grape leaves
- 1–2 lemons, thinly sliced to make about 20 slices
- 2 cups water

## For Yogurt Sauce:

- 2 cups plain non-fat yogurt
- 4 scallions, minced
- 1 clove fresh garlic, minced
- 1 teaspoon salt

## How to Prepare

1. Inside a skillet over moderate heat, add 1 tablespoon of olive oil, onions, and scallions; cook till soft and colorless.

2. Add rice and cook until grains are slightly browned, stirring constantly. Add garlic, cumin, pepper, and vegetable broth.

3. Lower heat to simmer, close, and cook until rice is tender and all liquid is absorbed. Allow rice to cool, then stir in fennel, dill, parsley, and mint. Set aside.

4. Drain grape leaves and cover with water; bring to a rolling boil. Blanch leaves for 1–2 minutes, drain, and allow to cool.

5. With leaf shiny side down, fill with rice mixture and roll starting at the stem and folding in the sides. Repeat until all 20 leaves are filled.

6. Line a heavy-bottomed pan with 10 of the unfilled grape leaves. Pack the rolled leaves in tightly side by side, seam side down. Top the rolled leaves with lemon slices and cover lemon slices with remaining unfilled grape leaves.

7. Mix together water and remaining olive oil and pour over grape leaf rolls. Place an object like a heavy plate on top of rolls to help hold them below the water level during cooking, and simmer for about 1 hour, checking to make sure they haven't boiled dry.

8. Withdraw pan from stove and allow to cool. Remove rolls from pan and chill. Serve chilled or at room temperature. Serve with yogurt sauce on the side as a dip.

**Yogurt Sauce:**

Mix together plain yogurt, scallions, garlic, and salt to taste. Chill until ready to serve

## 21.   Tomato and Garlic Bruschetta

Serving: 8 servings

### Ingredients

- 8 slices (½ thick) of a French baguette or a crusty whole grain bread
- 1 teaspoon extra virgin olive oil

- 1¼ cups chopped plum tomatoes
- 1½ teaspoons minced fresh garlic
- 1 teaspoon balsamic vinegar
- ½ teaspoon dried basil
- ¼ teaspoon non-caloric sweetener
- ¼ teaspoon freshly ground pepper

**How to Prepare**

1. Place slices of bread on a non-greased baking sheet.

2. Brush every slice with olive oil and bake in a small bowl for 3–4 minutes until golden brown.

3. Combine tomatoes, garlic, sugar, basil, sweetener and pepper in a small bowl.

4. Mix well and spoon mixture over slices of bread.

## 22. Tomato and Fresh Parmesan Cheese Bruschetta

Serving: 8 slices

**Ingredients**

- 8 slices (½ inch thick) of a French baguette or crusty whole grain bread 2
- cloves fresh garlic, finely minced
- 1 teaspoon extra virgin olive oil + more for brushing 1 small onion, diced
- 1 medium tomato, diced
- Pinch dried oregano, crumbled
- Pinch freshly ground pepper
- 2 tablespoons freshly grated Parmesan cheese

**How to Prepare**

1. Scantly brush slices of bread on both sides with olive oil, then toast.

2. Remove from oven and evenly distribute garlic on one side of bread. Rub garlic into bread with handle of knife and set aside; keep warm.

3. Heat teaspoon of olive oil in skillet, add onion, and lightly sauté until golden brown. Remove from heat. Preheat broiler.

4. Combine onion, tomato, oregano, and pepper; spread evenly over garlic bread and sprinkle with Parmesan cheese.

5. Place bread with Parmesan cheese under broiler for 1 minute until lightly browned.

Serve immediately.

## 23. Italian Crostini

Serving:  25 to 27 servings

**Ingredients**

- 1 French baguette, roughly 10–12 inches long, cut into ½ inch thick slices
- Extra virgin olive oil cooking spray
- 2½ teaspoons fresh garlic paste
- Salt and freshly ground pepper to taste
- Dry or fresh basil, parsley or chives.

**How to Prepare**

1. With a small amount of cooking oil, spray gently on both sides of each slice of bread.

2. Brush a side of each slice with a little amount of garlic paste, then sprinkle herb of choice over garlic. Season with salt and pepper.

3. Layer slices on a non-stick cookie sheet and layer them on the middle rack in a 375°F (190°C) oven for baking until slices are a light golden brown (about 3 to 5 minutes).

4. If needed, serve as is or add your favorite topping (smoked mozzarella, cut fresh tomatoes, chopped black olives, roasted garlic, etc.).

## 24.    Mushroom Crostini

Serving: 4 servings

**Ingredients**

- 1 (10–12 inch) loaf of crusty whole grain bread
- Olive oil cooking spray
- 1½ tablespoons trans-fat–free canola/olive oil spread 1 tablespoon extra virgin olive oil
- 3 tablespoons minced shallots
- 2 tablespoons freshly minced garlic
- 4 cups assorted mushrooms (such as crimini, shiitake, button, or portobello), sliced
- ½ cup sherry
- 1 tablespoon freshly chopped parsley
- 1 teaspoon freshly chopped thyme
- Salt and freshly ground pepper to taste
- Freshly grated Parmesan cheese for garnish (optional)

**How to Prepare**

1. Slice bread into 8 thick slices. Sprinkle gently slices with cooking oil on both sides and put them on a non-stick baking sheet.

2. Bake until the slices are golden brown and crisp. Allowing the spread of canola/olive oil to reach room temperature.

3. Heat olive oil in a big skillet, add shallots and garlic and cook until tender.

4. Add mushrooms and sherry to a mixture of garlic and cook until mushrooms are tender and most of the liquid has evaporated (stir gently to merge flavors during cooking).

5. Mix in canola / olive oil spread, parsley, thyme and salt and pepper to taste when mushrooms are soft.

6. Mix spoon mushroom on toasted slices of bread and sprinkle with scant amounts of Parmesan cheese, if desired.

## 25.    Antipasti

Serving: 10-15 servings

**Ingredients**

- Fruits (select whatever is in season), cut into manageable pieces
- Cheese
- Seafood

**How to Prepare**

1. Cheese: use soft and hard, and spicy and mild, cheese, leaving some in whole wedges and slicing or chunking others)

2. Seafood: try big to jumbo cooked shrimp, tails on but otherwise shelled; cooked calamari; steamed clams; mussels; smoked oysters)

3. Other products: try to include marinated artichokes, black and green olives of various size

4. Before adding everything to the platter, ensure all items are drained of liquid. Serve the antipasti with a tray of crunchy whole grain bread or sticks of bread.

# 26. Avocado Spread with Crusty Garlic Toast

Serving: 4 servings

## Ingredients

- 1 large ripe avocado, pitted and peeled
- ½ cup fresh cilantro leaves
- 1 clove fresh garlic, chopped
- 2 tablespoons minced scallions
- 1 tablespoon a freshly squeezed lemon juice
- 1 tablespoon extra virgin olive oil
- Salt and freshly ground pepper to taste
- 4 slices (½ inch thick) whole grain baguette
- Olive oil cooking spray
- ½ teaspoon garlic powder
- 1 tablespoon shredded Parmesan cheese
- 4 thin slices jalapeño pepper(optional)

## How to Prepare

1. Preheat water broiler. In a food processor, add avocado, coriander, garlic, scallions, lemon juice, olive oil, salt and pepper, and process until butter is smooth. Put aside.

2. Sprinkle cooking oil on both sides of each baguette slice, and put on a baking sheet covered with foil.

3. Sprinkle garlic powder and Parmesan cheese over the baguette tops.

4. Place the baking sheet under broiler slices around 6 inches and broil until slightly toasted.

5. Remove from heat, allow to cool, and cover with spreading avocado.

6. Complete with very thin jalapeño strips and serve.

# 27.  Baby Shrimp on Roasted Rye

Serving: 12 to 16 servings

## Ingredients

- ½ cup reduced-fat mayonnaise
- 2 tablespoons finely minced shallot
- 1 tablespoon finely chopped fresh parsley
- 1 teaspoon Dijon mustard
- ½ teaspoon chopped capers
- 16 slices cocktail-sized, thin rye bread
- Garlic/olive oil cooking spray
- 1 bag cooked salad shrimp, thawed

## How to Prepare

1. Scant splash 16 paper-thin lemon slices of freshly squeezed lemon juice.

2. Whisk the mayonnaise, shallot, parsley, mustard, and capers together in a small bowl.

3. Cover and refrigerate to mix flavors for no less than 1 hour. In the meantime, brush rye slices lightly with garlic/olive oil spray and toast to 300°F (150°C) in a toaster oven or oven until slightly crispy.

4. Remove from the oven and scatter over each slice of rye toast 1 teaspoon of mayonnaise mixture. Finish with 4 to 5 shrimps and a small lemon juice scatter. Add lemon slices to garnish.

# 28.  Hummus and Alfalfa Sprouts

Serving: 12 Servings

## Ingredients

- 12 large whole grain crackers

- 1½ cups hummus
- 12 slices low-fat cheddar cheese
- 12 tablespoons alfalfa sprouts
- Freshly ground pepper
- Lemon wedges for garnish

**How to Prepare**

1. Arrange the crackers in a dish.

2. Equally spread hummus over crackers.

3. Top with a slice of cheddar cheese, sprouts, and pepper sprinkling on each cracker.

4. Garnish platter with lemon wedges before enjoying by squeezing over crackers.

## 29.    Apple, Gorgonzola and Walnut Crostini

Serving: 24 servings

**Ingredients**

- 24 thin slices French bread
- Olive oil cooking spray
- 2 Granny Smith apples, cored and thinly sliced
- 8 oz. crumbled gorgonzola cheese
- 1 cup chopped walnuts

**How to Prepare**

1. Cover broiler to preheat.

2. Sprinkle bread slices lightly on both sides with a scant amount of cooking oil.

3. Place slices under broiler on both sides on a baking sheet and toast, turning once, until slightly brown.

4. Place 2 slices of apple on each piece of toast and remove from broiler. Finish with a mound of gorgonzola cheese on every piece.

5. Put pieces of walnut into cheese and return to broiler. Broil until cheese melts, while cheese and walnuts are browned lightly. When dry, serve.

## 30.  Avocado and Mango Salsa

Serving: 4 Servings

**Ingredients**

- ½ red onion, finely chopped
- 1 ripe avocado, peeled and cut into ½ inch cubes
- 2 ripe mangoes, peeled and cut into ½ inch cubes
- ½ jalapeño pepper, seeds removed and finely diced
- 2 tablespoons fresh cilantro, finely chopped
- Juice from 1 lime
- Salt and freshly ground pepper to taste

**How to Prepare**

1. In a dish, add the onion, avocado, mango, jalapeño, coriander and lime juice.

2. Blend well to bring ingredients together. To try, season with salt and pepper. Cover and cool to refrigerate. Use as fish topping or as chip dip.

## 31.  Bay Scallops with Smoked Paprika

Serving: 10 servings

## Ingredients

- 1½ tablespoons olive oil
- 1½ tablespoons trans-fat–free canola/olive oil spread
- 1 pound fresh bay
- scallops (about 100 scallops)
- Smoked paprika to coat
- 1 lemon, halved, one half to squeeze and the other thinly sliced for garnish
- 10 small wood skewers.

## How to Prepare

1. Heat olive oil and canola/olive oil spread over medium-high heat in a large heavy-bottom skillet.

2. Gently remove scallops and brush scallop tops with smoked paprika. Stir often as the scallops start browning.

3. Drizzle over half a lemon with freshly squeezed juice and steam for about 3 minutes or until cooked through. Don't overcook them.

4. Skewer 10 scallops on each skewer and squeeze over skewers to serve with thin slices of lemon.

## 32.    Caponata

Serving: 6 servings

## Ingredients

- 1 medium eggplant
- 1 heaping tablespoon sea salt
- 2 tablespoons extra virgin olive oil
- 1 medium yellow onion, chopped
- 2 cloves garlic, minced
- 1 medium red bell pepper, chopped

- 1 medium yellow bell pepper, chopped
- 6 fresh tomatoes, blanched and peeled, or 1 large can of tomatoes
- ½ teaspoon (or less) red pepper flakes (non-compulsory)
- 1 tablespoon red wine vinegar
- 2 teaspoon sugar
- 1 cup pitted and coarsely chopped black olives (not California style).
- ¼ cup capers, cleaned and drained
- 1 tablespoon a chopped fresh Italian parsley (flat-leaf )
- 1 tablespoon a chopped fresh basil (or 1 teaspoon dried)

## How to Prepare

1. Cut the eggplant into cubes that are dice sized.

2. Place in a colander and toss with sea salt. Place a paper towel over the eggplant and place the colander in the sink.

3. Cover with a plate or bowl to weigh down the eggplant (use a bowl if the colander is big and a plate does not put any weight on the eggplant.

4. Weigh the plate or bowl with something like a 1-pound tomato can. Allow the eggplant to drain into the sink for about 30 minutes.

5. Sprinkle a non-stick skillet with olive oil spray and heat over medium-high heat till it thickens and divide into a more or less homogenous mixture (it should look more like a sauce than a stir-fry), about 30 minutes, then keep cooking for another 30 minutes, stirring frequently to keep the caponata from burning and sticking to the skillet

6. Lastly, add the capers, olives, petersil and basil. Remove the caponata from the heat.

7. Let it cool to room temperature, then serve or store in the refrigerator in an airtight container for up to 3 days.

# 33.    Shish Kebab

Serving: 4 servings

**Ingredients**

**For the meat/fish marinade:**

- Get 1 tablespoon olive oil
- Get juice of a fresh lemon
- Get 1 minced garlic clove
- Get 1 teaspoon a crushed dried thyme.
- Get 1 teaspoon a dried cumin powder
- ½ teaspoon paprika
- ¼ teaspoon cayenne pepper
- A dash black pepper

**For the shish kebab:**

- A pound of any of lamb (for originality), beef tenderloin (if you cannot find or do not wish to eat lamb), cod or shrimp (for the coastal version) or a combination of the three, for variety
- 1 medium red onion
- 1 green bell pepper
- 1 red bell pepper
- 16 cherry tomatoes
- 4 cups fresh greens
- 4 pita loaves

**How to Prepare**

1. Merge all the ingredients for the marinade in a pot. Cut into cubes of bite size the meat or fish. Add the meat to marinade and mix. Close the lid and wait for at least 2 hours, or overnight.

2. Cut the bell peppers and the onion into bite-sized chunks. Fill one or two long skewers with onion, one or two long skewers

with bell peppers, and one or two long skewers with cherry to-matoes.

3. Place the meat / fish cubes marinated on long skewers.

4. Sprinkle grill or broiler pan with spray or canola oil for cooking.

5. Heat the grill or preheat broiler (any of the two)

6. Grill or broil meat or fish until it is cooked, rotating as required to cook evenly on all sides. Lamb and beef take about thirty minutes, cod and/or shrimp about fifteen to twenty minutes, or to the doneness needed. Include onion and pepper skewers to the grill or broiler roughly halfway through meat cooking time. Add tomato skewers during the final 5–10 minutes. Continue to watch meat and vegetables and remove from heat once all vegetables are cooked.

7. Certain individuals like and prefer their meat well done, also vegetables properly done, while some people like it less done. Wrap the pita loaves in foil over the last 5 minutes and put them on.

8. When cooking all meat and vegetables, remove meat from a plate and vegetables from a separate plate. As desired, fill every pita with meat, vegetables, and greens.

## 34.    White Beans with Cumin

Serving: 4 servings

**Ingredients**

- 1 can of white beans (navy beans, great northern beans, or any other white beans)
- 1 tablespoon natural cut off basil (or 1 teaspoon dried basil)
- ½ teaspoon cumin

- 1 teaspoon extra virgin oil

**How to Prepare**

1. Drain the beans into a colander, then rinse well. Place them in a dish.

2. Stir in basil, cumin, and olive oil. Leave it at room temperature.

The next day, these are great straight from the fridge, especially when paired with crisp, chilled, fresh greens.

In this dish, simply remove the olive oil to cut the calories and fat.

# CHAPTER 10
# MAIN AND SECOND COURSES RECIPES

## 35.    Mediterranean Chickpea Salad

Preparation time: 10 minutes

**Ingredients**

- ½ cup extra virgin olive oil
- ¼ cup white wine vinegar
- 1 tablespoon lemon juice
- 1 tablespoon freshly chopped parsley
- ¼ teaspoon red pepper flakes
- Kosher salt
- Freshly ground black pepper

**How to Prepare**

1. To make the salad, toss chickpeas, cucumber, bell pepper, red onion, olives and feta together in a large bowl. Season with pepper and salt.

2. Vinaigrette: Mix olive oil, vinegar, lemon juice, parsley, and red pepper flakes in a container fitted with a lid. Close the jar and shake, then season with salt and pepper until emulsified.

3. Dress up salad and serve with vinaigrette.

## 36.    Italian Chicken Skillet

Preparation time: 40 minutes

Serving: 4 servings

**Ingredients**

- 2 tablespoon extra virgin olive oil
- 1 lb. boneless skinless chicken breasts
- Kosher salt
- Freshly ground black pepper
- ½ onion, thinly sliced
- 2 bell peppers, thinly sliced
- 2 medium zucchini, sliced into half moons
- 2 cloves garlic, minced
- ½ teaspoon dried oregano
- 1 cup low-sodium chicken broth
- 1 (14 oz.) can of crushed tomatoes
- ¼ cup freshly torn basil

**How to Prepare**

1. Heat oil over medium-high heat in a large skillet. Season the chicken using salt and pepper and cook until golden and cooked through for about 8 minutes each side. Put on plate

2. Add the onion and pepper to the skillet and cook until tender for 5 minutes. Add the zucchini and cook until slightly charred for 3 minutes, then add the garlic and continue to cook for 1 minute until it is fragrant. Season it with oregano.

3. Bring the broth and the crushed tomatoes together, and simmer for 10 minutes. Return the chicken to the sauce for skillet and vegetable sauce. Until serving, garnish with basil.

# 37.    Mango Salsa Topped Halibut

Preparation time: 20 minutes

Makes 4 servings

### Ingredients for the Halibut

- 4 (4-6 oz.) halibut steaks
- 2 tablespoons extra virgin olive oil
- Kosher salt
- Freshly ground black pepper

### Ingredients for the Mango Salsa

- 1 mango (diced)
- 1 red pepper (finely chopped)
- ½ red onion (diced)
- 1 jalapeno pepper (minced)
- 1 tablespoon freshly chopped cilantro
- Juice of 1 lime
- Kosher salt
- Freshly ground black pepper

### How to Prepare

1. Preheat grill to medium-high and spray olive oil on both sides of the halibut. Season with salt and pepper, on both sides.

2. Grill the halibut for about 5 minutes per side and cook through each side.

3. In a medium bowl, combine all ingredients together and season well with pepper and salt to make the salsa. Serve over salsa with the halibut.

## 38.    Easy Greek Salad

Preparation time: 15 minutes

Serving: 4 servings

### Ingredients for the salad

- 1 pt. Grape or cherry tomatoes (halved)

- 1 cucumber, thinly sliced into half moons
- 1 cup halved kalamata olives
- ½ red onion, thinly sliced
- ¾ cup crumbled feta

## Ingredients for the dressing

- 2 tablespoons red wine vinegar
- ½ a lemon (juiced)
- 1 teaspoon dried oregano
- Kosher salt
- Freshly ground black pepper
- ¼ cup extra virgin olive oil

## How to Prepare

1. To make the salad, stir in a large bowl the tomatoes, cucumber, olives and red onion. Gently fold in the feta.

2. Combine the vinegar, lemon juice, and oregano, and season in a small bowl with salt and pepper. Gradually apply olive oil, whisk to blend. Drizzle up the dressing over the salad.

## 39.    Lemon Garlic Shrimp

Preparation time: 15 minutes

Serving: 4 servings

## Ingredients

- 2 tablespoons butter, divided
- 1 tablespoon extra-virgin olive oil
- 1 lb. medium shrimp, peeled and deveined
- 1 lemon, thinly sliced, plus juice of 1 lemon
- 3 cloves garlic, minced
- 1 teaspoon crushed red pepper flakes
- Kosher salt

- 2 tablespoons dry white wine (or water)
- Freshly chopped parsley, for garnishing

## How to Prepare

1. Melt 1 tablespoon butter and olive oil in a skillet over medium heat. Add the shrimp, the lemon slices, the garlic and the crushed red pepper flakes, and season with salt.

2. Cook by stirring regularly, approx. 3 minutes per side until the shrimp is pink and opaque.

3. Remove and stir the remaining lemon juice of butter and white wine. Season with salt before serving and garnish with parsley.

## 40.    Spicy Sole

Serving: 4 Servings

## Ingredients

- Spicy Pistachio Pesto
- 8 (3 oz.) fillets of sole
- Salt and freshly ground pepper to taste
- 1 cup water
- 1 cup dry white vermouth
- 1 tablespoon fresh lemon juice

## How to Prepare

1. Prepare the sauce for pesto and set aside. Cover with salt and pepper over the filets and roll with the toothpicks. Put it aside.

2. Bring the malt, vermouth and lemon juice to a boil; add the rolled filets, cover and poach for about seven minutes, until the meat turns white and the fish is cooked through.

3. Cut rolled fillets off skillet with a slotted spoon. Serve straight away in a plate and top with Spicy Pistachio Pesto. Serve whilst it's hot.

## 41. Spanish Paella with Saffron Rice, Seafood and Chicken

Serving: 8 servings

### Ingredients

- 2 pounds skinless, boneless chicken, cut into pieces
- Dash of freshly ground pepper
- ¾ teaspoon garlic salt
- ½ cup extra virgin olive oil
- ¼ pound lean boneless pork, cut into ½ inch cubes
- ½ cup chopped onion
- ½ medium red bell pepper, seeded and sliced
- ½ medium yellow bell pepper, seeded and sliced
- 1 large tomato, peeled and finely chopped
- 2 cloves fresh garlic, crushed
- 3 cups long-grain rice
- ½ teaspoon salt
- ¼ teaspoon ground saffron
- 6 cups water
- 1 cup frozen peas, thoroughly defrosted
- 12 medium shrimp
- 7 hard-shelled clams
- ½ pound garlic-seasoned smoked pork sausage

### How to Prepare

1. Steam shrimp in a little water until it's just pink, then put it by the side. Scrub the clams under running water then steam the clams in ample water to cover them. Extract from water with a slotted spoon when clams open and set aside.

2. In several places prick sausage with fork, put on heavy skillet, and cover with cold water.

3. Bring water to a boil and bring heat down to low. Simmer the sausages for about 15 minutes, uncovered. Drain the sausages well, then slice and set aside into ¼ inch round pieces.

4. Rinse the chicken properly, pat dry, and season with salt of pepper and garlic and heat ¼ cup olive oil in a large skillet, add the pieces of chicken and fry until crispy. Take the browned golden chicken from the skillet and put on paper towel-lined plate.

5. Add the pieces of sausage to the skillet, brown them quickly and drain on a plate lined with paper towels. Remove olive oil from skillet and use paper towels to dry skillet. Heat ¼ cup fresh olive oil into the same skillet until dry. Stir in pork cubes and easily brown.

6. Attach bell peppers, tomato, and garlic, onion, red and yellow. Cook the vegetables and meat continuously, stirring until tender and set aside

7. Add rice, salt, saffron, and 6 cups water in a large pot; bring to a boil and cover, stirring occasionally, until the rice is fluffy. Switch rice, shrimp and remaining milk, clams, bacon, chicken and pork cubes and vegetables to a casserole dish that is ready for the oven.

8. Sprinkle the peas over the mixture, put the saucepan on a 400°F (200°C) oven bottom rack and bake for twenty to thirty minutes or until liquid is absorbed. When the paella has cooked, remove it from the oven, cover it with clean kitchen towel, and let it stand for 5 minutes. Serve straightaway.

Note: The oven should be preheated 30 minutes prior to placing paella inside.

## 42.   Skewered Mediterranean Grilled Lamb and Vegetables

Serving: 4 serving

**Ingredients**

- 2 lemons (juiced)
- ⅓ cup extra virgin olive oil
- 1 clove fresh garlic, minced
- 1 tablespoon chopped mint
- Salt and freshly ground pepper to taste
- 1½ pounds lamb sirloin, cut into 1½ inch cubes
- 8 large bay leaves
- 8 fresh mushroom caps
- 8 small cherry tomatoes
- 1 big green bell pepper, seeded and cut into 1½ inch strips
- 2 small zucchinis, cut into 1 inch cubes
- 4 medium onions, quartered

**How to Prepare**

1. In a resealable plastic baggie, mix lemon juice, olive oil, garlic, mint and add salt and pepper to taste. Place in the refrigerator and marinate for at least 8 hours overnight.

2. Alternate the meat, bay leaves, and vegetables on 8 flat-bladed oiled skewers. Grill for about 15 minutes over hot coals, turning the skewers over several times.

3. This dish goes well with a chopped onion salad, cucumbers, tomatoes and parsley. For dressing, use lemon juice.

## 43.   Baked Stuffed Trout

Serving: 4 servings

**Ingredients**

- 3 tablespoons extra virgin olive oil
- 1 large onion, finely chopped
- 4 cloves fresh garlic, minced
- ⅔ cup plain breadcrumbs
- 1 lemon, juiced and rind-grated
- ⅓ cup seedless dark raisins, chopped
- ½ cup pine nuts
- 2 tablespoons chopped fresh parsley
- 1 tablespoon chopped fresh dill
- Salt and freshly ground pepper to taste
- ¼ cup egg substitute
- 4 (12 oz.) whole trout, scaled and gutted
- Olive oil cooking spray
- Lemon wedges for garnish

**How to Prepare**

1. Heat 2 spoonful's of olive oil in a skillet, add onion and garlic and cook until soft, then remove from heat. Mix breadcrumbs, rubbed lemon rind, raisins, pine nuts, parsley, dill, and salt and pepper in a large bowl; add garlic mixture and egg, then mix well. Fill each trout with mixture and put on an oil-sprayed, shallow baking pan in a single layer.

2. Make multiple diagonal slashes of lemon juice and drizzle remaining tablespoon of oil along the body of each fish. Bake for about 30–45 minutes at 375°F (190°C), or until the fish flakes. Serve warm, with lemon wedges to garnish.

## 44. Great Northern Beans and Chicken

Serving: 6 servings

**Ingredients**

- 2 (3 oz.) skinless, boneless chicken legs
- 2 (4 oz.) skinless, boneless chicken breasts

- 2 onions, chopped into large pieces
- 5 carrots, 1 sliced and cut the other 4 into large pieces
- 2 stalks celery, 1 sliced and the other cut into large pieces
- Olive oil cooking spray
- 2 cups canned low-sodium, fat-free chicken broth
- 4 cups canned Great Northern beans, drained and rinsed
- 2 tomatoes, peeled and chopped into large pieces
- ½ green bell pepper, chopped into large pieces
- 2 teaspoons fresh thyme
- 3 cloves fresh garlic, chopped
- 2 tablespoons chopped fresh parsley
- Salt and freshly ground pepper to taste

**How to Prepare**

1. Rinse the chicken and pat dry before spraying with the cooking oil. Put the chicken, half the onions, 1 sliced carrot and 1 sliced stalk of celery in a saucepan. Apply water to cover the chicken and cook until chicken is tender over medium heat. Drain, and set aside.

2. Lightly coat the bottom and sides of a large casserole dish with the spray and add chicken, 2 cups broth and beans. Add remaining pieces of carrot and celery and tomatoes, remaining onion, green bell pepper, thyme, garlic, parsley and salt and pepper to the casserole. Bake for 45 minutes, until it simmers.

3. Serve while it's hot

## 45. Bouillabaisse

Serving: 4 servings

**Ingredients**

- 2 teaspoons extra virgin olive oil
- 2 leeks, white and green parts, thinly sliced

- 3 cloves fresh garlic, minced
- 2 cups freshly chopped tomatoes
- ¼ cup dry white wine
- 1 tablespoon tomato paste
- 1 tablespoon freshly chopped parsley
- ½ teaspoon dried thyme
- 2 bay leaves
- ⅓ teaspoon crushed saffron
- ⅛ teaspoon fennel seeds
- 10 oz. fresh firm cod, cut into 1½ inch chunks
- 2 (6 oz.) fresh lobster tails, quartered
- 16 littleneck clams, scrubbed
- 3 oz. orzo, cooked and drained

**How to Prepare**

1. Combine olive oil, leeks, and garlic in a large saucepan over medium-high heat; cook for about 3 minutes, stirring occasionally. Add tomatoes, 1½ cups water, wine, tomato paste, parsley, thyme, bay leaves, fennel seeds, and saffron. Stir to combine.

2. Boil the mixture and stir periodically. Add cod, lobster, and clams; bring to boil again. Reduce heat, covered, to low and simmer for six to eight minutes. Fish and lobster are to be cooked until they are finished and clams until they open.

3. Remove the bay leaves and spoon the cooked orzo into 4 bowls of soup; ladle Bouillabaisse over orzo and serve.

## 46. Spicy Broccoli Rabe with Penne Pasta

Serving: 4 servings

**Ingredients**

- 2 pounds fresh broccoli rabe, cleaned, trimmed, and cut into 1 inch pieces

- 1 pound whole wheat penne pasta
- 3 tablespoons extra virgin olive oil
- 5 cloves fresh garlic, thinly sliced
- 1 medium white onion, chopped
- 2 oz. anchovy fillets, drained
- ¼ teaspoon crushed red hot pepper flakes
- Salt and freshly ground pepper to taste
- Freshly grated Romano cheese for garnish (optional)

**How to Prepare**

1. Boil water and salt in a large saucepan. Add the rabe broccoli and cook for about 5 minutes, until the stems are tender. Move the broccoli to a colander for drain with a slotted spoon. Return the broccoli broth to a boil, and add pasta.

2. Cook until tender and rinse, reserving ¼ cup water for pasta. Return the pasta to a bowl and keep warm. Heat olive oil in a large skillet, then add the garlic and onion; sauté until golden for about 2 minutes. Remove pepper flakes and anchovies, stirring for about 1 minute.

3. Attach rabe broccoli and cook for another 5 minutes, until warm. Add pasta and enough reserved pasta liquid to the broccoli rabe mixture to moisten slightly; toss until well combined. Season with salt and pepper. Garnish with Cheese Romano. Serve warm.

## 47.    Grilled Citrus Salmon with Garlic Greens

**Ingredients**

- ¼ cup orange marmalade
- 2 tablespoons fresh lime juice
- 2 tablespoons fresh lemon juice
- ¼ cup low-sodium soy sauce

- 3 teaspoons grated orange rind
- 4 (3 oz.) salmon fillets
- 2 teaspoons extra virgin olive oil
- 2 teaspoons minced fresh garlic
- 2 (10 oz.) bags fresh spinach
- Small amount of olive oil to rub on fish
- Salt and freshly ground pepper to taste
- 1 teaspoon fresh garlic, mashed to rub on fish
- 1 heaping tablespoon capers, drained
- 1 tablespoon balsamic vinegar
- 4 scallions, white and light green parts, thinly sliced (2–3 inch lengths)

**How to Prepare**

1. Whisk marmalade, lime and lemon juices, soy sauce and orange rind together; pour over the fillets and marinate in a refrigerator for 30 minutes. Prepare broiler with grill or preheat in the oven.

2. Heat the olive oil over medium-high heat in a heavy skillet; add the garlic and spinach, one bag at a time, and sauté, stirring frequently until the spinach is wilted (about 2 minutes).

3. Reduce heat to very low, to retain warmth. Combine the olive oil, salt and pepper, garlic crushed, and capers. Rub the paste into Salmon steaks on both sides.

4. Grill the fish on each side for 2–2½ minutes, or broil 3–4 inches from the flame. Set aside birds. Remove the spinach from heat and mix with vinegar; break on 4 plates equally. Add salmon grilled fillet to spin bed.

## 48. Sicilian Style Linguine with Eggplant and Roasted Peppers

Serving: 6 servings

## Ingredients

- 2 large yellow bell peppers
- 1 small eggplant, peeled and cut into ½ inch cubes
- 2 tablespoons extra virgin olive oil
- 2 tablespoons minced fresh oregano
- 2 tablespoons capers
- 4 teaspoons minced fresh garlic
- 1 (35 oz.) can peeled plum tomatoes
- ½ teaspoon crushed red hot pepper flakes
- Salt and freshly ground pepper to taste
- 1 pound linguine
- 1 cup shredded fresh basil leaves
- ¾ cup grated Romano cheese

## How to Prepare

1. Fill broiler with preheat. Halve bell peppers and cut seeds. Cut each half into strips and place skin side up on baking sheet, broil until blackened. Set the oven to 400°F (200°C). Toss the eggplant cubes with 1 tablespoon of olive oil and put the cubes on a baking pan in one layer.

2. Bake for about 25 minutes, until it is very tender and browned, turning to bake evenly once. Heat 1 tablespoon of olive oil over medium-high heat in a large skillet; add oregano, capers, and garlic, and sauté until garlic is lightly golden.

3. Garnish with eggplant, bell peppers, tomatoes and milk, hot pepper flakes, and salt and pepper. Cover, reduce heat, and simmer, stirring occasionally, for about 15 minutes. Cook the pasta in boiling water, drain and place it back in the pot. Pour over pasta sauce, add basil and mix gently. Sprinkle with Cheese Romano and drink.

# 49.    Chicken and Eggplant

Serving: 8 servings

## Ingredients

- 2 medium eggplants, peeled and cut into 1½ inch cubes
- ½ cup + 2 tablespoons extra virgin olive oil, divided
- 3 pounds skinless, boneless chicken
- 2 large onions, chopped
- 4 cloves fresh garlic, chopped
- 4 large tomatoes, peeled, seeded, and chopped
- 2 teaspoons Thick Pomegranate Molasses
- 3 tablespoons freshly squeezed lemon juice
- Salt and freshly ground pepper to taste
- 2 tablespoons finely chopped fresh parsley
- 1 teaspoon mixed spices

## To make mixed spices combine

- 2 teaspoons allspice
- 1 teaspoon ground cinnamon
- 1 teaspoon ground cloves
- 1 teaspoon fresh cilantro
- 1 teaspoon ground cumin
- ¼ teaspoon freshly ground pepper

## How to Prepare

1. Generously salt the eggplant parts and let drain in a colander for about 30 minutes (this drives its bitter juices). Rinse pieces under running cold water after 30 minutes, squeeze pieces gently with hands to remove excess moisture, and pat dry with paper towels.

2. Heat ½ cup olive oil over medium heat in a large, heavy skillet. Add half of the pieces of the eggplant and sauté, often turning un-

til golden brown. Transfer pieces (using a slotted spoon) into paper towels to drain and soak up excess oil. Repeat with the remaining eggplant, if necessary add more olive oil.

3. Pour olive oil out of the skillet, let the skillet cool down, and wipe it clean. Rinse bits of chicken under cold water and pat dry with paper towels. Place chicken in skillet with 2 tablespoons of olive oil and sauté, turning on all sides to brown evenly. Transfer parts into plate. Pour off all but three tablespoons of skillet drippings.

4. At medium heat, add the onions and sauté until golden brown. Stirring. Add tomatoes, Thick Pomegranate molasses, lemon juice and salt and pepper to taste, add the garlic and mixed spices and sauté for about 30 seconds. Return chicken and any juices from plate to pan, spooning over bits of tomato mixture. Bring to boil and turn the heat to low. Cover and simmer for approximately 45 minutes or until chicken is tender. Stir in the sautéed parsley and eggplant, cover and simmer for another 10 minutes. Change to taste seasonings. Serve with a pasta side dish (optional).

## 50.    Spicy Whole Wheat Meal Capellini with Garlic

Serving: 4 servings

### Ingredients

- 8 oz. whole wheat capellini pasta
- ¼ cup extra virgin olive oil
- 4 cloves fresh garlic, chopped
- 1 teaspoon diced red hot pepper
- Salt and freshly ground pepper to taste
- Grated Pecorino or Parmesan cheese (optional)

### How to Prepare

1. Put the pasta into water and bring it to a boil. Cook the pasta until it is done. Drain the pasta and restore it to the pot with little olive oil to keep the pasta from bonding. Put this aside

2. Sprinkle the garlic, and hot pepper over medium heat (for about 1–3 minutes). Warm olive oil in a heavy pot over medium heat. Pour in pasta and sprinkle with parmesan cheese if necessary. Add salt and pepper to taste.

## 51.    Broiled Red Snapper with Garlic

Serving: 4 servings

### Ingredients

- 3 tablespoons lemon juice
- 1 cup dry white wine
- 1 chilli pepper, chopped
- 1 whole red snapper (about 2–2 ½ pounds), scaled and gutted
- 3 cloves fresh garlic, finely chopped
- 2 tablespoons extra virgin olive oil
- Olive oil cooking spray
- 2 tablespoons chopped fresh oregano
- 2 tablespoons chopped fresh parsley
- Salt and freshly ground pepper to taste
- Lemon wedges for garnish

### How to Prepare

1. In a shallow pan, marinate the cleaned shrimp with 1 tablespoon lemon juice, wine, chilli pepper and 1 clove garlic for 1 hour in the refrigerator.

2. Preheat the broiler. Whisk the remaining lemon juice, olive oil, and salt and pepper together. Rub mixture inside and outside of

fish. Place the fish on a broiler pan sprayed with oil and sprinkle with the oregano.

3. Broil the fish for about 10 minutes, regularly basting with a mixture of olive oil and turning once, until golden brown. In the meantime, blend the remaining garlic and parsley together. Sprinkle the parsley mixture over the cooked fish and serve hot, garnished with wedges of lemon.

## 52.    Pasta with Pine nuts and scallops

Serving: 4 Servings

### Ingredients

- 8 oz. tagliatelle or fettuccine
- 4 tablespoons extra virgin olive oil
- 3 cloves fresh garlic, finely chopped
- 1 leek, white part only, thinly sliced
- 10 pitted black olives, halved
- ¼ cup pine nuts
- 12 large sea scallops, halved
- Salt and freshly ground pepper to taste
- 2 tablespoons chopped fresh basil
- Parmesan cheese, finely grated, for garnish (optional)

### How to Prepare

1. Boil the water, add the pasta, and cook the pasta until al dente.

2. Remove from heat, drain pasta, and return to the pot, sprinkling with little olive oil to prevent pasta from sticking together. Set it aside.

3. Heat olive oil in a skillet while pasta is cooking, add garlic and leek, and cook until soft but not brown.

4. Remove olives and pine nuts and sauté until light browning of pine nuts. Add the scallops and cook until opaque. Season with salt and pepper.

5. Apply to pasta and mix scallops and pan juices. Sprinkle with basil and, if needed, garnish with Parmesan cheese.

## 53. Spicy shrimp with angel hair pasta

Serving: 4 servings

**Ingredients**

- 8 oz. angel hair pasta
- 1½ pounds medium shrimp, peeled and deveined
- 1 teaspoon low-calorie baking sweetener
- ¼ teaspoon salt
- 1 tablespoon chilli powder
- ½ teaspoon ground cumin
- ½ teaspoon ground coriander
- ½ teaspoon dried oregano
- 1 tablespoon + 1 teaspoon extra virgin olive oil
- Lime wedges for garnish

**How to Prepare**

1. Boil water, add pasta, and cook pasta until al dente.

2. Remove from heat, drain pasta, and return to pot, drizzling with scant amount of olive oil to keep pasta from sticking together. Set aside.

3. Sprinkle shrimp with sweetener and salt. Combine chilli powder, cumin, coriander, and oregano, then lightly coat shrimp with spice mixture.

4. Heat one tablespoon of olive oil in a big non-stick skillet over medium-high heat. Add half of the shrimp and sauté about 4 minutes, or until cooked.

5. Remove cooked shrimp from pan and repeat procedure with 1 teaspoon olive oil and remaining shrimp.

6. Divide cooked pasta into 4 servings, top with shrimp and pan sauce, and garnish with lime wedges. Serve immediately.

## 54.    Fruit glazed salmon with couscous

Serving: 4 servings

**Ingredients**

- ¾ pound couscous
- 2 cups canned low-sodium, fat-free chicken broth, heated
- ½ cup apricot jam
- 3 tablespoons thinly sliced scallion
- 2 tablespoons prepared horseradish
- 1 tablespoon white wine vinegar
- ½ teaspoon salt (divided)
- 4 (6 oz.) salmon fillets, 1 inch thick, skinned
- ¼ teaspoon freshly ground pepper
- 2 teaspoons extra virgin olive oil

**How to Prepare**

1. Clean an oven-safe dish and put the couscous in the platter.

2. Pour in the chicken broth and let sit until the couscous is tender and the liquid is absorbed for 10 minutes.

3. Mount the dish in a low-temperature oven and keep warm until ready to serve.

4. Meanwhile, stir well with a whisk and mix apricot jam, scallion, horseradish, vinegar, and ¼ teaspoon salt.

5. Sprinkle with remaining salt and pepper to the salmon fillets. Heat olive oil over medium-high heat, in a large non-stick skillet.

6. Add salmon and boil for 3 minutes. Turn the salmon with half the apricot mixture and brush.

7. Wrap the handle of the skillet with foil and bake the salmon in the skillet for 5 minutes at 350°F (180°C), or until the fish flakes.

8. Extract salmon from the oven and brush with remaining apricot mixture. Serve with a couscous for each fillet.

## 55.    Pasta primavera with shrimp

Serving: 4 servings

### Ingredients

- 1 pound whole wheat penne pasta
- ½ cup canned low-sodium, fat-free chicken broth
- Extra virgin olive oil to drizzle + 2 teaspoons
- 2 dozen medium shrimp, cleaned, peeled, and deveined
- 1½ cups broccoli florets
- 1 medium red bell pepper, thinly sliced
- 1 cup halved button mushrooms
- 1 cup frozen peas
- ½ cup sliced scallions
- 4 cloves fresh garlic, minced
- 1 oz. (2 tablespoons) dry white wine
- 2 tablespoons freshly grated Parmesan cheese

### How to Prepare

1. Bring water to boil, add pasta, and cook pasta until al dente.

2. Remove from heat, drain pasta, and return to the pot, drizzling with little olive oil to prevent pasta from sticking to each other. Set aside.

3. Heat ¼ cup broth, 2 teaspoons of olive oil, and shrimp in a large non-stick skillet; cook until the shrimp are pink. Remove shrimp with a slotted spoon and set aside.

4. Add broth, broccoli, red bell pepper, mushrooms, peas, scallions, and garlic to the skillet. Cook for 4–5 minutes, stirring frequently, until the vegetables are tender, and the liquid is mostly absorbed.

5. Add wine, simmer for about 1 minute, and add shrimp to the mixture of vegetables. Place penne pasta in a large serving bowl and add remaining olive oil to toss.

6. Add a mixture of vegetables; toss well to mix. Sprinkle with Parmesan cheese.

## 56.    Turkish Mussel Stew

Serving: 6–8 Servings

**Ingredients**

- 1 cup dry white wine
- 1 cup water
- 6 dozen mussels, scrubbed and de bearded (discard any open mussels)
- 2 tablespoons extra virgin olive oil
- 1 medium onion, peeled and sliced
- 1 leek, white part only, sliced
- 6 cloves fresh garlic, coarsely chopped
- 4 large tomatoes, peeled and diced
- 2 large white potatoes, peeled, sliced about ¼ inch thick
- 2 medium carrots, cleaned and chunked
- Pinch of saffron
- 2 bay leaves
- Salt and freshly ground pepper to taste
- ¼ cup finely chopped fresh flat leaf parsley

## How to Prepare

1. Combine wine, water, and mussels in a large, heavy casserole dish. Cover mussels with pan and steam until they open (around 7–10 minutes).

2. Remove the mussels from the liquid and discard any unopened. Set aside the liquid of the mussel.

3. Take the mussels from the shells and add a small amount of liquid to keep them damp. Strain and set aside remaining liquid mussel using cheesecloth.

4. Add olive oil and sauté gently onion, leek, and garlic into a clean saucepan until tender, then add tomatoes and cook for another 1–2 minutes.

5. Remove slices of potato, carrots, saffron, bay leaves and strained liquid mussels; cover with pan and cook over medium-low heat until vegetables are tender (about 30 min).

6. Attach the mixture to the mussels and continue cooking until all is fully heated; attach salt and pepper to taste.

7. Stir in parsley and remove from heat. Serve hot while serving.

## 57.    Spicy Julienned Sweet Potato fries

Serving: 4 servings

### Ingredients

- 1 pound sweet potatoes, peeled and julienned
- 1 tablespoon olive oil
- 1 tablespoon light brown sugar
- 1 teaspoon salt or to taste
- ½ teaspoon chilli powder
- Pinch of cayenne pepper
- ¼ teaspoon ground cinnamon

### How to Prepare

1. Preheat oven to 450°F (230°C) and lay out a large foil baking sheet.

2. Combine the potatoes, olive oil, brown sugar, salt, chilli powder, cayenne and cinnamon in a big, resealable plastic baggie.

3. Toss well from the bag to cover and wash. Arrange potatoes on baking sheet in a single layer and bake for approximately 15 minutes.

4. Switch over the potatoes and bake for another 15 minutes, or until crispy.

## 58.    Italian Broccoli

Serving: 4 servings

### Ingredients

- 2 large stalks of broccoli, stems detached and heads cut in half
- 1 cup Italian dressing mix of your choice
- ⅓ cup dry white wine
- Salt and freshly ground pepper to taste
- ½ cup grated Parmesan cheese (optional)

### How to Prepare

1. Place the broccoli heads cut sideways in a wide rimmed baking dish in a single layer. Whisk Italian dressing and wine together and pour over heads of broccoli.

2. Lift each head so that liquid also covers the cut sides of the heads.

3. Cover with plastic wrap on the baking dish and put in the refrigerator to marinate for at least 1 hour.

4. Place the heads in a saucepan after marinating, pour marinade over the heads and steam until tender.

5. Remove the heads from the remaining liquid and serve hot, sawn to taste with salt and pepper, and sprinkle with Parmesan cheese.

## 59.    Roasted Baby Artichokes and Parmesan Cheese

Serving: 4 servings

**Ingredients**

- 4 numbers (9 oz.) of boxes frozen baby artichokes hearts
- 2 cups canned reduced sodium and fat-free chicken broth
- 4 cloves fresh garlic, coarsely chopped
- Salt and freshly ground pepper to taste
- 1 cup panko breadcrumbs
- ½ cup grated Parmesan cheese
- Melted trans-fat–free canola/olive oil spread, to drizzle

**How to Prepare**

1. Preheat oven to 350°F (180°C).

2. Place the artichoke hearts, broth, garlic, salt and pepper in a large pot. Take to a gentle boil and cook until the core is tender for about 3 minutes.

3. Drain to preserve pieces of garlic and artichoke through a wide sifter.

4. Spread the artichokes and garlic evenly, top with a layer of breadcrumbs in a rimmed oven-safe casserole dish, then sprinkle on Parmesan cheese.

5. Place in the oven and bake and crumbs are a golden brown when heated through. Serve hot with a sprinkling of melted canola/olive oil

## 60.    Sautéed Kale and Spinach with Mushroom and Tomato

Serving: 4 servings

### Ingredients

- 4 tablespoons olive oil, divided
- 4 tablespoons chopped fresh garlic
- 3 bunches fresh kale, leaves only
- Crushed red hot pepper flakes to taste
- One (9 oz.) bag of fresh baby spinach
- ¼ cup water, if required
- Salt and freshly ground pepper to taste
- ½ large white onion, chopped
- 2 (8 oz.) containers fresh white button mushrooms, halved
- 10–15 grape tomatoes
- 2 tablespoons fresh garlic paste blend

### How to Prepare

1. Add 2 tablespoons of olive oil and garlic in a large skillet over medium-high heat, and sauté until soft and fragrant.

2. Add the kale, a handful at a time, and hot pepper flakes and cook until kale is wilted, stirring frequently. Remove baby spinach and keep cooking until wilted. If required, add water to keep it moist. Season to taste, using salt and pepper.

3. Reduce to very low heat and keep warm. Add the remaining 2 tablespoons of olive oil to a separate skillet over medium heat.

4. Add onion, chestnuts, grape tomatoes, and paste for garlic. Allow to cook.

5. Keep stirring, until the mushrooms are soft, and the tomatoes start breaking down. Season with salt and pepper.

6. Mix tomato mixture plus spinach mixture and return heat to a simmer, stirring for about 2 minutes to combine ingredients and flavors. Serve while hot.

## 61.    Boiled Red Fresh Beets

Serving: 4 servings

### Ingredients

- 8 medium red beets, unpeeled
- Water to cover beets
- Salt and freshly ground pepper, to taste
- Butter-flavored cooking spray (optional)

### How to Prepare

1. Wear disposable gloves or kitchen gloves to avoid staining hands since the skins and juices of fresh red beets stain the skin and clothing.

2. Remove the stems from the beets, and the root ends. Wash the beets, rub the skins gently to extract as much dirt as possible from the beets.

3. In a large pot, put unpeeled beets, and cover with water. Boil over medium to high heat until the beets are tender.

4. Remove from heat and drain the juice through a strainer; retain if you like the beet root juice. Place the beets in the pot under running cool water and gently remove the skins from the beets, again using beet stains with gloves.

Season with salt and pepper and a butter mist, if desired, and serve.

## 62.    Oven Roasted Potato Wedges

Serving: 6 servings

**Ingredients**

- 1½ pounds russet potatoes, clean and cut lengthwise into wedges
- ¼ cup olive oil
- ½ teaspoon smoky paprika
- ¼ teaspoon garlic salt or to taste
- Cayenne pepper to taste
- Freshly ground pepper to taste

**How to Prepare**

1. Preheat oven to 450°F (230°C).

2. In a big, resealable plastic baggie, combine the potato wedges, olive oil, paprika, garlic salt, cayenne, and pepper.

3. Toss well with olive oil and seasonings to coat both sides of potatoes.

4. Remove from the bag, place wedges on a foil-lined baking sheet in a single layer and bake, stirring once after 10–15 minutes, until the wedges are golden and crispy (about 25–30 minutes).

## 63.    Couscous with Turnips and Greens

Serving: 4 to 6 Servings

**Ingredients**

- 2½ cups fat-free chicken broth (canned) with low sodium

- 3 tablespoons olive oil, divided
- 1½ cups pearl couscous
- 1 bunch baby turnips plus greens, peeled and quartered
- ½ teaspoon cumin seeds
- 2 cloves fresh garlic, minced
- ½ medium-sized white onion, finely cut
- Salt and freshly ground pepper to taste

**How to Prepare**

1. Add the broth and 1 tablespoon of olive oil in a medium sauce-pan and bring to boil. Stir in the couscous, cover and let stand.

2. Cut the heads off greens and wash well both heads and greens, remove any brown or wilted seeds. Cut greens into roughly 1 inch bits and cut turnips into halves. Set aside the vegetables and the turnips.

3. On medium-high heat, apply remaining olive oil to a large skillet. Add the cumin and cook until fragrant for 1 minute.

4. Put the garlic and continue cooking for about 1 minute, until soft and fragrant. Add onion and stir, then cook until smooth.

5. Add turnips, cover pan and cook, stirring occasionally, until crispy tender.

6. Cook till greens wilt. Fluff couscous with a fork and transfer to a large bowl, add cooked vegetable mixture, fluff it all over again and serve immediately.

## 64. Grilled Polenta plus Cheddar Cheese and Sundried Tomatoes

Serving: 6 Servings

**Ingredients**

- 6 cups water Salt to taste
- 1¾ cups yellow cornmeal
- 1½ tablespoons chopped fresh oregano
- 1½ tablespoons chopped fresh basil
- 3 tablespoon trans fat–free canola/olive oil spread
- 6 oz. reduced-fat shredded cheddar cheese
- 6 sundried tomato slices

**How to Prepare**

1. Boil water in a big saucepan, then add salt.

2. Little by little, whisk in cornmeal. Reduce heat to low, and cook a mixture of cornmeal until it thickens, often stirring for about 15 minutes.

3. Remove from heat, add oregano, basil and spread canola / olive oil and stir until the mixture has melted.

4. Move to a lightly oiled 7 inch baking dish, spreading thinly to around ¾ inch thickness. Refrigerate for at least 2–3 hours, until cold and solid. Invert polenta onto a clean surface when firm, then cut into pieces of 2x2 inches.

5. Set barbecue grill to medium heat. Spray the polenta on both sides with olive oil and sear until golden brown on each side (about 3 minutes).

6. Remove from heat and sprinkle with cheddar cheese when dry, and top with a sundried slice of tomato. Serve straightaway.

## 65.    Broccoli with Almond and Olives

Serving: 4 servings

**Ingredients**

- 2 tablespoon extra virgin oil (olive)
- 1 clove fresh garlic, minced
- 2 teaspoon grated lemon zest

- ½ tablespoon lately squeezed lemon juice
- 12 pitted Kalamata olives, chopped
- ⅛ teaspoon pounded red hot pepper flakes
- ¼ cup toasted almonds, chopped
- 1 head fresh broccoli (about 1 pound), florets only, blanched
- 1½ tablespoon fresh parsley, chopped
- Salt and freshly ground pepper to taste

**How to Prepare**

1. In a big bowl, mix the olive oil, garlic, lemon zest, lemon juice, olives, hot pepper flakes, and almonds.

2. To taste, add blanched broccoli florets, parsley, salt and pepper. Throw in the coat and serve warm.

## 66.     Broiled Avocado Halves and Cheddar Cheese

Serving: 4 servings

**Ingredients**

- 2 ripe-but-firm avocados, halved and pitted, with the skin on
- ¼ cup reduced-fat, shredded, extra-sharp cheddar cheese
- 1 small jalapeno pepper, finely minced (about 1 teaspoon)
- Salt and freshly ground pepper to taste
- 1 tablespoon fresh lime juice
- 1 lime, quartered, for garnish

**How to Prepare**

1. Preheat the broiler.

2. Place the avocado halves on a cut side-up, lined baking sheet.

3. Mix cheddar cheese, jalapeno, salt and pepper, and lime juice in a small mixing bowl. Divide the cheese mix between the tops of the halves of avocado.

4. Place the baking sheet 3–4 inches under heat and broil for about 3–5 minutes or until the cheese bubbles and start to brown. Serve warm halves with lime wedges.

## 67.    Kale with Orange Mustard Dressing

Serving: 8 Servings

**Ingredients**

- 1 tablespoon olive oil
- 2 bunches fresh kale, stems detached, leaves slice to bite sized pieces
- 2 radishes, sliced thin
- 1 avocado, deseeded, peeled, and chopped
- For Dressing:
- 2 large oranges, peeled, pith detached, and segments split up
- 2 tablespoon grainy mustard
- ¼ cup extra virgin oil
- 1 teaspoon chopped fresh thyme leaves
- Salt and freshly ground pepper to taste

**How to Prepare**

1. Heat the olive oil over moderate heat in a large skillet.

2. Attach the kale, a handful at a time, and sauté until wilted, always stirring.

3. Switch from dressing and dressing to serving cups, add radishes, avocado, orange pieces left over.

4. To paint the kale mixture, split into 8 parts and serve warm.

## 68.    Baked Potato Fingers plus Shallots and Fresh Herbs

Serving: 4 servings

**Ingredients:**

- 4 large-sized Yukon Gold potatoes (about 1½ pounds)
- 2 tablespoon olive oil
- 2 large shallots, finely minced
- 1 tablespoon finely chopped fresh sage leaves
- 1 tablespoon finely chopped fresh rosemary
- Salt and freshly ground pepper to taste
- Olive oil cooking spray

**How to Prepare**

1. Preheat oven to 375°F (190°C).

2. Scrub the potato skins with a brush of vegetables, and pat dry. Split the potatoes lengthways in half. Cut each half into 4 slices in lengthwise direction.

3. Combine the olive oil, shallots, basil, rosemary, salt, and pepper in a small bowl.

4. Stir to blend. Spray cooking oil to a shallow baking sheet.

5. Arrange potato fingers on baking sheet in a single layer and brush them generously with shallot-herb mixture. Place in the oven and roast for 40 minutes, after about 20 minutes turning once. Roast until browned and tender to the fingers. Switch off oven and serve.

# 69.    Pass the Peas Please

Serving: 4 servings

## Ingredients

- 2 tablespoon olive oil
- 1 white onion, chopped
- 2 cloves fresh garlic, minced
- 16 oz. fresh or frozen peas, thawed
- ½ cup canned less sodium, fat-free chicken broth
- Salt and newly ground pepper to taste
- Pinch of sugar (optional)
- Butter spray

## How to Prepare

1. Heat olive oil inside a skillet over moderate heat.

2. Add onion and garlic and sauté until it is soft, nearly 4–5 minutes.

3. Add peas, broth, salt, pepper, and sugar, if you wish. Close and cook until peas are tender. Serve hot alongside a spritz of butter spray.


# 70.    Great Corn on the Cob

Serving: 4 servings

## Ingredients

- 4 teaspoon trans-fat–free canola/olive oil spread, melted
- Salt with newly ground pepper to taste
- 4 ears fresh corn, husks and silk detached
- 24 large fresh basil leaves

## How to Prepare

1. Heat oven to 450°F (230°C).

2. Mix canola/olive oil spread and salt and pepper in a bowl.

3. Brush buttery mix on corn to coat entire ear. Set every ear in heavy tinfoil.

4. Put 3 basil leaves on the bottom and 3 over the top of each ear.

5. Bend tinfoil over ears and twist ends to seal. Place foil-covered ears on a baking sheet. Bake for 15 minutes or until tender.


## 71.   Garlicky Swiss Chard

Serving: 6 servings or 3 cups

### Ingredients

- 2 bunches of Swiss chard (about 1½ pounds each), cleaned and trimmed
- 3 tablespoon extra virgin oil (olive)
- 6 cloves of fresh garlic, minced
- ½ cup canned less sodium, fat-free chicken broth
- ¼ teaspoon hot cherry peppers, finely minced
- ½ teaspoon salt or to taste
- ¼ teaspoon freshly ground pepper

### How to Prepare

1. Rinse greens well and cut ribs and stems into 2 inch pieces. Set aside. Break leaves into roughly 2 inch pieces.

2. Heat olive oil in a large heavy-bottomed skillet; add garlic and sauté until golden brown, stirring constantly.

3. Add chard ribs and stems, broth, and hot peppers and cook until almost tender. Add leaves in bunches, stirring to wilt. Stir in salt and pepper. Cook covered, until tender and liquid is evaporated, stirring often.

# 72.    Crispy Tender Ratatouille

Serving: 8 servings

## Ingredients

- 2 large eggplants, rinsed and cut in 1½ inch cubes
- 3 red of bell peppers
- ¾ cup extra virgin olive oil
- 2 large chopped onions
- 8 cloves newly produce garlic, minced
- 4 small zucchinis, cut to 1½ inch cubes
- 4 big ripe tomatoes, cored and dice
- 1 cup dry red wine
- 1 tablespoon capers, rinsed and drained
- 1 or 2 pinches of crushed red-hot pepper flakes or to taste
- Salt and freshly ground pepper to taste
- Freshly chopped basil for garnish (optional)
- Pitted black olives for garnish (optional)

## How to Prepare

1. Place eggplant cubes in a bowl with salt and cover with water. Place heavy plate inside bowl to weight down cubes, submerging them in brine. Set aside for 1½–2 hours.

2. Roast red bell peppers under broiler in oven until skins turn black and are easy to remove. Peel off skins and cut peppers into long strips. Set aside.

3. Heat ¼ cup olive oil in a large skillet over medium-low heat, add onions and garlic, and cook until soft. Do not brown.

4. Add roasted pepper to mixture. Drain eggplant cubes and pat dry with paper towels. Add another ¼ cup olive oil to skillet, return to medium heat, and sauté eggplant cubes until golden

brown (15 minutes). Add zucchini to skillet and cook, adding more olive oil if needed.

5. When zucchini is cooked, add tomatoes, lowering heat slightly; stir in wine and simmer until wine is evaporated and mixture turns to a jam consistency (about 20 minutes).

6. Stir in capers and hot pepper flakes and combine all vegetables with tomato sauce.

7. Use a slotted spoon to stir but don't break up vegetables. Add salt and pepper to taste. Before serving, add basil and olives, if desired.

## 73.    Broccoli with Fresh Garlic

Serving: 4 to 6 servings

### Ingredients

- 10–12 fresh broccoli spears, and roughly 6 inches long
- 3 cups canned low-sodium, fat-free chicken broth
- 3 tablespoon extra virgin olive oil
- 2–3 cloves of freshly crushed garlic.
- 2 tablespoon freshly chopped parsley
- Salt to taste
- Pinch of freshly ground pepper to taste

### How to Prepare

1. Cook spears in a big skillet of chicken broth until a bit under-cooked (almost 7 minutes). Test using a fork; do not overcook.

2. Empty out water and set aside. Heat olive oil in a large skillet over medium-high heat; add garlic and sauté until golden brown.

3. Include broccoli, parsley, and salt and pepper to taste. Turn spears several times, mixing well with seasonings, olive oil, and garlic. Serve immediately

## 74. Asparagus with Fresh Garden Herbs

Serving: 8 servings

**Ingredients**

- 1 pound of asparagus, tough ends detached
- 1 tablespoon finely chopped fresh parsley
- ½ tablespoon finely chopped fresh basil
- ⅛ teaspoon freshly ground pepper
- 3 tablespoon trans-fat–free canola/olive oil spread, melted
- 2 Italian plum tomatoes, seeded and chopped
- 2 tablespoon shredded Parmesan cheese

**How to Prepare**

1. Steam asparagus for 3–5 minutes until it is crispy tender. Drain well and put on a serving platter.

2. Incorporate parsley, basil, pepper, and canola/olive oil spread.

3. Drizzle combination on top of the asparagus, sprinkle on tomatoes and Parmesan cheese, and serve.

## 75. Couscous, Tomatoes and Black Beans

Serving: 4 to 6 servings

**Ingredients**

- 1½ cups canned low-sodium vegetable broth
- 1 cup couscous
- 1 tablespoon extra virgin olive oil
- 2 cloves of fresh garlic, minced
- ¼ cup fresh lemon juice
- ¼ teaspoon freshly ground pepper
- 1½ cups canned black beans, rinsed and drained
- 4 large plum tomatoes, chopped
- ½ cup red onion, finely chopped
- Fresh parsley, finely chopped for garnish

**How to Prepare**

1. In a saucepan, boil broth. Stir in couscous, take it out from heat, close, and let stand till liquid is taken in.

2. In a small skillet over medium heat, include olive oil and garlic and sauté until golden brown. Take away skillet from heat, include lemon juice and pepper, and combine ingredients through.

3. Transfer couscous to a big serving bowl. Fluff grains with fingers to separate. Add in garlic mixture, black beans, tomatoes, and onion; stir carefully to mix.

4. Garnish with parsley and serve.

## 76. Garlic Rice

Serving: 4 servings

**Ingredients**

- ½ tablespoon extra virgin olive oil
- 4 cloves of fresh garlic, minced
- 1 cup basmati long-grain rice
- 2 cups canned low-sodium, fat-free chicken broth
- ¼ cup grated Parmesan cheese

- 2 tablespoon chopped fresh parsley
- 3 jumbo cloves of roasted fresh garlic, cut into small piece
- Salt and freshly ground pepper to taste
- Fresh chopped parsley or cilantro for garnish

**How to Prepare**

1. Heat olive oil and sauté fresh garlic in a skillet till golden brown.

2. Boil rice and chicken broth, close tightly, reduce heat to simmer, and cook till liquid is taken.

3. Remove rice from heat and add olive oil and sautéed garlic, Parmesan cheese, parsley, roasted garlic, and salt and pepper to taste; toss well.

4. Garnish with parsley or cilantro and serve.

## 77.     Greek Rice

Serving: 4 servings

**Ingredients**

- 1 cup short-grain rice
- 2 cups canned low-sodium vegetable broth
- 1 tablespoon extra virgin olive oil
- 2 teaspoons minced fresh garlic
- 2 tablespoons finely chopped onion
- 5 oz. fresh spinach, cleaned and chopped
- ¼ teaspoon dried oregano
- Salt and freshly ground pepper to taste
- ¼ cup crumbled feta cheese
- 1 tablespoon lemon juice

**How to Prepare**

1. Bring rice to boil, cover tightly, reduce heat to warm, and cook until liquid is absorbed.

2. Heat olive oil over medium-high heat while rice is cooking, and sauté garlic and onion until golden.

3. Reduce heat to medium; add a little spinach at a time to allow wilting while mixing in garlic.

4. Include in the oregano, salt and pepper to taste when spinach is wilted.

5. Remove from heat the spinach mixture and add the cooked rice, feta cheese and lemon juice.


## 78.   Chilled Stuffed Pasta Shells

Serving: 4 servings

### Ingredients

- 1 cup (canned) hearts of palm, chopped and well drained
- 1 cup chopped zucchini
- 2 cloves fresh garlic, finely minced
- 8 large pitted black olives, chopped
- 2 tablespoons chopped fresh parsley
- 2 tablespoons + 2 teaspoons extra virgin olive oil
- 4 teaspoons freshly squeezed lemon juice
- Salt with a freshly ground pepper to taste
- 12 jumbo pasta shells, cooked al dente and drained
- 4 cups mixed salad greens

### How to Prepare

1. In a large bowl, add palm hearts, zucchini, garlic, olives, and parsley.

2. For vinaigrette, whisk together olive oil, lemon juice, salt and pepper.

3. Add 2 tablespoon vinaigrette to bowl of vegetables, then mix gently. Stuff the shells with a mixture of vegetables, cover and refrigerate until well chilled.

4. Refrigerate the remaining vinaigrette

5. Divide greens into 4 equal portions to serve, top each serving with 3 stuffed shells and drizzle with the rest of the vinaigrette.

## 79.    Classic Spinach and Pine Nuts

Serving: 4 servings

### Ingredients

- ¼ cup golden raisins
- 4 tablespoons pine nuts
- 2 tablespoons extra virgin olive oil
- 4 cloves fresh garlic, chopped
- 1½ (10 oz.) bags fresh spinach, cleaned
- Fresh lemon juice
- Extra virgin olive oil to taste
- Salt and freshly ground pepper to taste

### How to Prepare

1. Put the raisins into a bowl and close it with water to boil. Let stand for about 10 minutes, until the raisins plump then drain well.

2. Toast pine nuts in a skillet over medium heat, stirring constantly for about 1–2 minutes. Take off heat and set aside.

3. Heat up olive oil in a big skillet. Stir in garlic and sauté 1–2 minutes, until golden. Add a little spinach at a time until it all gets wilted (about 3–5 minutes), stirring constantly.

4. Pour the raisins over the spinach, then mix. Move spinach to a serving dish with a slotted spoon and scatter the pine nuts over top.

5. Serve immediately or add fresh lemon juice and olive oil and salt and pepper to taste, if served at room temperature.

## 80.    Roasted Peppers

Serving: 4 servings

### Ingredients

- 4 large red bell peppers
- 2 cloves fresh garlic, peeled and sliced
- 4 tablespoons extra virgin olive oil
- Salt and freshly ground pepper to taste

### How to Prepare

1. Clean peppers and pat to dry. Place peppers under a broiler 1–2 inches from heat on a moderately hot grill or on a rack, turning often until the skin is charred and blistered. It takes about 15–20 minutes to char the whole face. Bring out from grill or broiler and set aside to cool the peppers.

2. Rub off blackened skins when it's cool enough to handle.

3. Cut each pepper in half, detach stalks and seeds and cut into strips of ½ inches. Layer strips in a bowl and stir in garlic, olive oil and salt and pepper.

4. Toss and place it aside for 30 minutes before serving.

# 81.   Orzo with Feta Cheese and Broccoli Florets

Serving: 8 Servings

## Ingredients

- 2 cups broccoli florets
- 3 cups canned low-sodium, fat-free chicken broth
- 8 oz. orzo (about 1 cup)
- 6 oz. feta cheese

## How to Prepare

1. Cook broccoli florets in boiling water until they are soft. Set aside, drain and keep warm.

2. Boil chicken broth in a saucepan, reduce heat, add orzo, and cook until it absorbs the liquid. Stir enough so as not to smoke.

3. Fluff orzo with fork and put feta cheese, stirring to blend. Move orzo and top with broccoli florets to serving platter.

# 82.   Zesty Lemon Swiss Chard

Serving: 4–6 Servings

## Ingredients

- 1¼ pounds Swiss chard, cleaned and trimmed
- 2 tablespoons fresh lemon juice
- 1½ teaspoons extra virgin olive oil
- 1 tablespoon lemon pepper seasoning
- Salt to taste
- ½ cup golden raisins
- 2 tablespoons pine nuts

## How to Prepare

1. Shred Swiss chard in thin strips and put in a big dish.

2. Combine lemon juice, olive oil, salt and lemon pepper seasoning; mix well with whisk. Drizzle over chard and toss.

3. Add the pine nuts and raisins, and toss. Let stand for 15 minutes before serving.

## 83.   Saffron Rice

Serving: 4–6 Servings

### Ingredients

- 3–4 cups canned low-sodium, fat-free vegetable broth
- 1 tablespoon extra virgin olive oil
- 4 tablespoons chopped shallots
- 2 cloves fresh garlic, minced
- 1 cup short-grain rice
- 1 cup dry white wine
- ¼ teaspoon crushed saffron threads
- ½ teaspoon dried thyme
- Salt and freshly ground pepper to taste

### How to Prepare

1. Boil the broth and then reduce heat.

2. Warm the olive oil in a large skillet, add shallots and garlic, then sauté until soft (about 5 minutes).

3. Add rice and start to sauté, continuously stirring to keep the mixture from burning.

4. Put wine, saffron and thyme, stirring constantly, scraping any brown bits from the pan.

5. Slowly add simmering broth when the wine is consumed, stirring constantly as broth is absorbed and rice has become tender (about 15–20 minutes).

6. It is likely that some of the broth is left over. Season with salt and pepper.

# CHAPTER 11
# SNACKS RECIPES

## 84.    Chocolate Bites

Serving: 24 Bites

**Ingredients**

- ½ cup unsweetened cocoa powder
- Pinch of salt
- ¼ cup low-calorie baking sweetener, divided
- 3 large eggs, whites only
- ¼ teaspoon cream of tartar
- 1 teaspoon pure vanilla extract
- 1 tablespoon confectioner's sugar (optional)

**How to Prepare**

1. Preheat oven to 400°F (200°C).

2. Line a baking sheet with foil. In a small bowl, sift together cocoa powder, salt, and ⅛ cup sweetener. Set aside.

3. In a large bowl, combine egg whites and cream of tartar. Beat using an electric beater until peaks form. Slowly add in remaining sweetener and beat until meringue forms stiff peaks.

4. Fold in cocoa mixture and vanilla extract. Drop rounded teaspoons of mixture 1 inch apart onto baking sheet.

5. Bake for 25 minutes and remove from oven.

6. Lightly dust with confectioner's sugar, if desired, and serve.

## 85. Cinnamon and Flaxseed Wafers

Serving: 12–16 Wafers

**Ingredients**

- 3 cups ground flaxseed
- 2 tablespoons ground cinnamon
- 6 packets non-caloric sweetener
- 1½ cups water
- Canola oil cooking spray

**How to Prepare**

1. Preheat oven to 350°F (180°C). In a large bowl, mix together flaxseed, cinnamon, and sweetener. Stir to blend ingredients. Add water and keep stirring until well blended. Set aside.

2. Lay parchment paper or waxed paper down on a flat surface. Form mixture into palm-sized balls and roll out to ⅛ inch thickness with a rolling pin lightly sprayed with cooking oil.

3. Cut rolled-out mixture into desired size for wafer pieces and place on a baking sheet lined with foil and gently sprayed with cooking oil.

4. Bake for about 30–35 minutes until crispy. Remove from heat and allow to cool before serving


## 86. Tuna Steak with Green Sauce

Serving: 4 servings

**Ingredients**

- 4 (6 oz.) grilled or broiled tuna steaks
- ½ cup walnut pieces
- ½ cup chopped cilantro
- ½ cup chopped fresh basil

- 1 teaspoon an extra virgin olive oil
- ½ cup chicken broth (maybe a little more or less)

**How to Prepare**

1. Select tuna steaks about 1 inch thick, and grill or broil for about 5 minutes on each side, or until fish flakes easily.

2. If the serving size is too big, split the fish parts in half then keep the other half as a nourishing treat the next day.

3. In the bowl of a meal processor, merge walnuts, cilantro, basil, olive oil, and half the chicken broth. Process it.

4. Put remaining chicken broth 1 tablespoon at a time, processing between additions till sauce is thick but can be poured.

5. Drizzle over hot or cold tuna steaks.

## 87. Falafel with Tomato – Cucumber Relish

Serving: 4 servings

**Ingredients**

- 1 medium onion, coarsely chopped
- ¼ cup parsley, minced
- 2 cloves garlic, minced
- ½ teaspoon ground cumin
- 1 teaspoon dried oregano
- 1 tablespoon a fresh lemon juice
- Salt with a newly ground black pepper to taste
- 1 cup dry whole-wheat breadcrumbs
- 1 big egg, gently beaten with a fork
- Olive oil cooking spray
- Tomato-Cucumber Relish (recipe follows)

## How to Prepare

1. In a food processor well suited with the metal blade, process the garbanzo beans, onion, parsley, garlic, cumin, and oregano until smooth.

2. Season to taste plus the lemon juice, salt, with pepper. Stir in ½ up of the bread atom and egg. Spread leftover breadcrumbs on a plate.

3. Using your hands, form the bean mixture into 16 round balls, rolling each ball in the breadcrumbs to coat. Set the balls on wax paper until you have them all coated.

4. Spray a large non-stick skillet with the cooking spray and put over moderate heat till hot. Include falafel balls and cook, stirring, till balls are browned, close to 10 minutes.

5. Put in order 4 falafel balls on each plate, and serve using the Tomato-Cucumber Relish, or stuff fresh greens and falafel in pita halves, topping with relish.

## 88.    Tomato-Cucumber Relish

Serving: 4 servings

### Ingredients

- ½ cup chopped tomato
- ½ cup chopped cucumber
- ⅓ cup non-fat pure yogurt
- ¼ teaspoon dried mint (optional)
- Salt with a newly ground black pepper to taste

### How to Prepare

Inside a small bowl, combine the tomato, cucumber, yogurt, and mint leaves; season to taste with salt and pepper.

## 89.  Swordfish Steak with Tomato-Caper Sauce

Serving: 4 servings

**Ingredients**

- 4 grilled or broiled swordfish steaks (about 6 oz. each)
- 2 big tomatoes, seeded and chopped (you can peel them if you like, but it isn't necessary (to seed, quarter tomatoes then squeeze the seeds out into the sink, then chop)
- 1 clove of minced garlic
- ¼ cup capers
- 1 teaspoon a dried tarragon (or basil or oregano, depending on which you prefer)
- Sea salt and black pepper to taste
- 1 teaspoon an extra virgin olive oil

**How to Prepare**

1. Cook swordfish steaks about 1 inch thick, and grill or broil for approximately 5 minutes on each side, or until fish flakes easily.

2. The sauce is quick and simple. If the serving size seems too large, divide the fish portions in half and keep the other part as a delicious treat the next day.

3. Mix tomatoes, garlic, capers, tarragon (crush dried herbs with your palms before adding to release flavour), salt, pepper, and oil.

4. Serve at room temperature over swordfish steaks (or any other fish, or chicken).

## 90.  French Cassoulet

Serving: 8 servings

**Ingredients**

- ½ pound of boneless pork tenderloin, smoked or cooked, and cut into small dice sizes
- ½ pound of a lean smoked sausage, preferably from Europe, cut into ½ inch slices
- 1 tablespoon extra virgin olive oil
- 1 big yellow peeled and chopped onion
- 1 big red bell pepper, chopped
- 2 cloves garlic, minced
- Four (15 oz.) cans navy beans, drained and rinsed
- One (14½ oz.) can diced tomatoes
- 1 teaspoon dried thyme
- 1 cup chicken broth
- Sea salt and black pepper, to taste
- 2 cups whole-grain breadcrumbs
- 1 additional teaspoon extra virgin olive oil

## How to Prepare

1. Heat the oven beforehand to 350°F (180°C).

2. Place pork and sausage inside a casserole or crock pot. Set aside.

3. Heat the olive oil in a medium size skillet over moderate heat for about 5 minutes.

4. Add the onion, red bell pepper, and garlic. Sauté, stirring often, till onions and pepper are soft but not browned, about 10 minutes. Put into casserole dish or an earthenware pot.

5. Include beans, tomatoes, thyme, and chicken broth to casserole dish or crock pot and stir all ingredients to form a mixture.

6. Spread the breadcrumbs over the cassoulet and drizzle with the left-over teaspoon olive oil.

7.In the casserole, bake uncovered until topping browns and filling is thick and bubbly, about 90 minutes. Or cook in an earthenware pot on low for 6–8 hours (in the crock pot, the topping won't brown the way it does in the oven, but the cassoulet still tastes delicious!).

## 91.   Paella Valencia

Serving: 8 servings

**Ingredients**

- 2 tablespoons extra virgin olive oil
- 1 whole chicken, cut into pieces
- ½ pound chorizo or spicy Italian sausage
- 2 onions, peeled and chopped
- 1 leek, chopped (white part only)
- 2 stalks celery, minced
- 3 cloves garlic, minced
- 2 red bell peppers, seeded and chopped inside thin strips
- 1 teaspoon ground cumin
- Pinch of saffron
- 2 cups white rice
- 2 cups chicken broth
- 1 (15 oz.) can chopped tomatoes
- 1 (15 oz.) can light red kidney beans, rinsed and drained
- 1 cup green peas
- 12 oz. peeled medium shrimp

**How to Prepare**

1. In a large non-stick skillet over medium heat, heat the oil for about 5 minutes.

2. Rinse chicken pieces and pat dry. Add chicken to the pan and sauté till chicken is golden brown. Remove to a plate and place aside.

3. Without wiping the pan, add the chorizo or other sausage to the pan, and sauté until fully cooked, about 10 minutes. Remove to a bowl and set aside.

4. Again, without wiping the pan, add onion, leek, celery, garlic, and red pepper. Sauté over moderate heat until vegetables are soft but not brown, about 5 minutes. Add cumin and saffron. Stir to combine.

5. Add uncooked rice and stir until rice is coated with oil and spices and thoroughly incorporated with the vegetables. Slowly pour chicken broth into rice mixture. Stir in tomatoes with their juice, kidney beans, and peas.

6. Pour the entire mixture into a large casserole or oven-safe Dutch oven. Arrange chicken pieces and shrimp on top of casserole in an attractive design.

7. Cover casserole or Dutch oven and bake for 45 minutes. Take out from the oven and let it sit for 10 minutes, or until rice has absorbed all the liquid.

## 92.    Almond Walnut Linguini

Serving: 4 servings

**Ingredients**

- 12 oz. dried linguine
- 1 tablespoon olive oil
- 1 cup chopped almonds
- 1 cup chopped walnuts
- 2 cloves garlic, minced
- 1 tablespoon fresh basil, minced, or 1 teaspoon dried basil
- 6 anchovy filets that is well chopped, or ½ teaspoon sea salt
- ¼ cup grated Parmesan cheese

**How to Prepare**

1. Cook linguine based on package directions, until al dente.

2. While cooking the linguine, toss olive oil, almonds, walnuts, garlic, basil, anchovies or salt, and cheese in a large bowl.

3. When pasta is done, drain, rinse, and instantly include to nut mixture. Toss to combine and serve right away.

## 93. Mediterranean Salad Sandwich with Harissa

Serving: 4 servings

**Ingredients**

- 1 (16 inch) baguette, divided into 4 pieces, each piece is halved longitudinally
- 2 cups salad greens
- Harissa, to taste (look recipe under, and never forget, this condiment can be very spicy, depending on the type of chillies you use to make it)
- Leftover fish and vegetables, such as:
- Cooked whitefish
- Cooked tuna
- Cooked salmon
- Cooked shrimp
- Sliced boiled potatoes
- Potato salad
- Cucumber slices
- Chopped tomatoes
- Relish, chutney, or salsa
- Chopped hard-boiled eggs
- Sliced red onion

**How to Prepare**

Spread in baguettes plus harissa. Top every sandwich using 1/2 cup salad greens and leftover fish and vegetables. Enjoy!

## How to make the Harissa

- ½ pound dried chillies, medium or hot or a mixture, depending on your preference
- 10 cloves garlic, peeled
- 1 teaspoon sea salt
- ½ cup caraway seeds
- 1 teaspoon a ground cumin
- 1 tablespoon an extra virgin olive oil, plus extra to cover the harissa for storage

## How to Prepare

1. Get rubber gloves for the safety of your hands (and anything they touch) from the hot chillies, pull off the stems and gently tap the sides to shake out the seeds.

2. Discard stems and seeds. Place the chillies in a large bowl. Pour hot water over the chillies to cover and set aside for approximately 30 minutes.

3. Put garlic cloves inside a food processor and process till minced.

4. In a smaller spice grinder or a well-cleaned coffee grinder, grind the salt, caraway seeds, and cumin until the caraway seeds are lower to the consistency of coarsely ground black pepper.

5. Pour this mixture into the food processor.

6. Add the drained, softened chillies (discard soaking water), and 1 tablespoon of oil. Process till the combination forms a paste.

7. Store in a smaller bowl or crock closed up using olive oil. Replenish olive oil anytime you use more harissa.

Serving: 6 to 8 servings

## Ingredients

- 1 medium onion, chopped
- 2 cloves garlic, minced
- 2 medium carrots, scraped and shredded
- 1 small stalk of celery, finely chopped
- 3 tablespoons an extra virgin olive oil
- 4 oz. extra lean ground beef or lean ground pork
- 1 (28 oz.) canned tomatoes with juice
- 2 tablespoons tomato paste
- 2 tablespoons chopped fresh Italian (flat-leaf) parsley
- 1 bay leaf
- ½ cup dry red wine or water
- 1 pound spaghetti, linguine, or vermicelli
- Freshly grated Parmesan cheese (optional)

## How to Prepare

1. In a large saucepan over moderate heat, sauté the onions, garlic, carrots, and celery in the olive oil. When the onions are translucent but not brown, add the ground beef.

2. Break up the meat with a wooden spoon and cook until brown. Stir in the tomatoes, tomato paste, Italian parsley, bay leaf, and the wine, if you are using it.

3. Lower the heat and simmer about 30 minutes, until thick but not dry. (If the sauce gets too dry, include more water, a little at a time, to reach desired consistency.).

4. Meanwhile, cook the pasta in boiling water and add salt to it. According to the package directions, until al dente (tender but firm).

5. Drain and restore the pasta to the warm pan (do not return to the hot burner). Just before serving, add the sauce and toss well.

6. Sprinkle grated Parmesan cheese over top if desired.

## 95. Seafood Risotto

Serving: 6 to 8 servings

**Ingredients**

- 10 large shrimp, peeled and divided into bite-sized pieces
- ½ pound crabmeat or lobster meat, divided into small chunks
- 2 tablespoon an extra virgin olive oil
- 3 cloves garlic, minced
- 1 large finely chopped onion
- 1 carrot, peeled and finely chopped
- 1 medium stalk of celery, minced
- ½ cup red bell pepper, finely chopped
- ½ cup green bell pepper, finely chopped
- 6 cups chicken or vegetable broth
- 2 cups uncooked Arborio rice
- ½ cup chopped fresh Italian (flat leaf) parsley
- ¼ cup freshly grated Parmesan cheese

**How to Prepare**

1. In a large non-stick saucepan over moderate heat, gently sauté the seafood in the olive oil. Stir for about five minutes.

2. Take out the seafood and put onto a paper towel. Without wiping the pan, add the garlic, onion, carrot, celery, and bell peppers to the pan. Sauté the vegetables until they are tender but not brown, about 10 minutes. In the meantime, set the water or broth on the stove to simmer.

3. Add the raw rice to the oil-vegetable mixture and mix to coat the rice with the oil, fully incorporating the vegetables.

4. Then begin to add the simmering broth, ½ cup at a time, letting each addition become almost completely absorbed by the rice and vegetables before adding the next ½ cup.

5. When the rice is tender and the mixture is looking like a sauce, stop adding broth (even if you haven't added it all) and stir in the cooked seafood.

6. Take off of the heat and stir in the Italian parsley and Parmesan cheese. Serve immediately.

## 96.    Eggplant Parmesan

Serving: about 6 to eight servings

**Ingredients**

- 1 finely chopped, small onion
- 2 cloves garlic, minced
- 2 tablespoons extra virgin olive oil
- One 28 oz. can chopped tomatoes
- 2 medium firm and fresh eggplants (weighing about 1 pound each)
- ¼ teaspoon sea salt
- ½ cup flour
- 2 large eggs, gently beaten
- 1 cup dried whole-grain breadcrumbs
- 1 pound of mozzarella cheese (choose part-skim to save on calories)
- 1 cup freshly grated Parmesan cheese
- 1 tablespoon chopped fresh Italian (flat leaf) parsley

**How to Prepare**

1. Heat the oven beforehand to 400°F (200°C). Prepare the tomato sauce: In a medium size skillet over a moderate heat, sauté the onion and garlic into 2 tablespoon the oil till the onion is colorless but not brown.

2. Include the diced tomatoes and stir to combine. Simmer carefully for 15 to 20 minutes, until the sauce thickens slightly. Take it away from heat. Meanwhile, rinse and slice the eggplants into thin slices of at most ¼ inch thick. (You may peel it if you wish, but it isn't necessary.)

3. Dip the eggplant slices in the flour, then into the egg mixture, then into the breadcrumbs to coat. In a large non-stick skillet, heat left over 2 tablespoons of olive oil until a bread crumb sizzles on contact.

4. Fry the eggplant slices rapidly, till tender and golden. Empty out on paper towels on a wire rack and sprinkle with the sea salt. Slice the mozzarella cheese into thin slices.

5. Coat a 9 by 13 inch baking pan with ½ cup the tomato sauce.

6. Then layer left over ingredients as follows: one-third of the eggplant slices, one-third of the remaining sauce, half the mozzarella slices, one-third of the eggplant slices, one-third of the sauce, half the grated Parmesan cheese, remaining eggplant, remaining sauce, remaining mozzarella, remaining Parmesan. Top with the chopped fresh parsley.

7. Bake 40 minutes at 400°F (200°C), remove from the oven, and allow to sit for at almost 15 minutes before cutting into squares and serving.

(Note: For a reduced fat variation, halve the amounts of mozzarella and Parmesan cheeses.)

# CHAPTER 12
# DESSERT RECIPES

## 97.  Fresh Fruit and Nut Platter

At the end of a Mediterranean meal, a platter of seasonal fresh fruits and different types of nuts is often served alone or in a mixed. Good fruits to try to include are bananas, kiwi, figs, dates, strawberries, grapes, peaches, plums, pears, melons, apples, pomegranates, currants and oranges with mandarins.

## 98.  Strawberry and Poached Pears

Serving: 4 Serving

**Ingredients**

- 4 large ripe Anjou or Bartlett pears, peeled and cored
- 2 tablespoons fresh lemon juice
- ½ cup red wine (not cooking wine)
- 1½ cups water
- 2 tablespoons low-calorie baking sweetener
- 1 cinnamon stick
- 1 teaspoon freshly grated orange rind
- ½ teaspoon freshly grated lemon rind
- ¼ teaspoon cloves, ground
- Fresh mint leaves for garnish

**For Strawberry Sauce:**

- 1 pint fresh strawberries, cleaned and sliced
- 3 tablespoons non-caloric sweetener
- 1 teaspoon Grand Marnier liqueur

## How to Prepare

1. Cut off the bottom of the pears so they can lie flat in a saucepan.

2. Brush most of the lemon juice into the pears.

3. Combine the wine, water, sweetener, cinnamon, orange rind, lemon rind, and cloves into a saucepan.

4. At medium heat, bring to a boil, reduce heat, and simmer for 5 minutes. Stir in pears, cover, and poach until tender for 20 minutes. Let the pears remain in fluid until cold.

5. Refrigerate until prepare for serving. Place pears on dessert plates when serving, and drizzle with a small amount of strawberry sauce. Top with mint leaf.

### Sauce:

Place strawberries in a bowl and sprinkle with Grand Marnier and sweetener. Let them stand for 1 hour at room temperature. Combine or process until purée, then refrigerate to chill sauce.


## 99.    Figs in Plain Yogurt

Serving: 4 Serving

### Ingredients

- 16 small figs
- 1½ cups red wine
- 2 tablespoons honey
- ¼ teaspoon ground cinnamon
- 2 cups plain low-fat yogurt
- Non-caloric sweetener, as desired
- Finely chopped fresh mint for garnish

### How to Prepare

1. Slice on one side the transparent skins of the figs. In a large saucepan, combine wine, honey, and cinnamon and bring the mixture to boil.

2. Reduce for 10–15 minutes to simmer, add figs, and simmer.

3. Remove from heat and let figs dry naturally for 5–10 minutes . Remove skins from the figs and mash.

4. Combine the mashed figs with yogurt, and mix well; if desired, add sweetener. Refrigerate well until chilled. Divide the yogurt mix into 4 bowls for dessert. Sprinkle with basil.

## 100.    Honey Mousse Delight

Serving: 6 Servings

### Ingredients

- ⅓ cup honey
- 2 teaspoons freshly grated orange rind
- 12 oz. part-skim ricotta cheese
- 2½ cups halved fresh strawberries
- 2½ cups fresh blackberries
- ¼ cup fresh orange juice
- 3 tablespoons non-caloric sweetener
- 2 tablespoons finely chopped walnuts

### How to Prepare

1. Using a medium size bowl, mix the honey, orange rind, and ricotta cheese. Cover and cool until chilled.

2. Combine the berries, fruit, and sweetener, toss gently and let stand 5 minutes before covering and chilling again.

3. When well chilled, spoon ⅓ berry mix (divided equally) into 6 serving bowls and top each with a mixture of about ¼ cup ricotta.

4. Divide the remaining fruit mixture into 6 servings, then sprinkle cheese and walnuts over the top before serving.

## 101. Spice Cake

Serving: 9 (1 inch wide) serving

**Ingredients**

- ½ teaspoon anise seed
- ¾ cup water
- ½ cup honey
- ½ cup low-calorie baking sweetener
- ½ teaspoon baking soda
- 3 cups unbleached white flour
- ⅛ teaspoon cinnamon
- ¼ teaspoon fresh grated nutmeg
- Pinch of salt
- ⅛ cup chopped orange mixed with lemon peels
- Olive oil spray

**How to Prepare**

1. Bring anise seed covered with water to a boil in a medium saucepan. Add honey and sweetener and whisk until both are dissolved.

2. Remove from heat the mixture and add baking soda.

3. In a large bowl, sift the rice, spices, and salt. Add lemon and orange peels. Strain liquid from anise seeds and mix the seeds into dry ingredients, constantly stirring.

4. Beat until the mixture is smooth, then pour over sprayed 9x5x3 inch and the baking pan is floured. Bake in the oven at 350°F (180°C) for 1 hour or until cake just starts shrinking from the sides of the pan.

5. Remove from the oven and slightly allow to cool. Serve warm or cold.

## 102.  Peach Marsala Compote

Serving: 6 Servings

**Ingredients**

- Canola oil cooking spray
- 12 fresh peaches
- 6 cups water
- ¾ cup low-calorie baking sweetener
- ½ cup Marsala wine
- ½ teaspoon ground cinnamon
- ½ teaspoon vanilla extract
- ½ teaspoon freshly grated nutmeg

**How to Prepare**

1. Sprinkle a 2 quarter baking dish generously with cooking oil.

2. Blanch the peaches for 20 seconds in boiling water, then cut the skin while keeping under cold running water. Pit pitches and slice.

3. Add peaches, sweetener, sugar, cinnamon, vanilla extract and nutmeg to a baking platter and bake in the oven at 350°F (180°C) for about 45 minutes to 1 hour. Serve warm, or at room temperature.

## 103.  Sautéed Peaches or Nectarines with Maple Syrup

Serving: 2 Servings

**Ingredients**

- 2 teaspoons canola oil
- 2 ripe peaches or nectarines, pitted, skinned, and sliced
- 2 tablespoons pure maple syrup
- Dash of ground cinnamon
- Dollop of plain yogurt per serving

**How to Prepare**

1. In a skillet, heat canola oil over medium-high heat, and sauté peaches or nectarines until golden, around 1–2 min.

2. Stir in maple syrup when golden and allow for a slight thickening of syrup.

3. Serve warm using a dollop of yogurt and a sprinkling of ground cinnamon.

## 104.  Sweet Mango Mousse

Serving: 6 Serving

**Ingredients**

- 1¼ cups water
- 1 cup couscous
- 4 tablespoons non-caloric sweetener
- ¾ cup fresh orange juice
- 2 tablespoons orange-flavored liqueur
- 1 large ripe mango
- 1 cup light whipping cream, well chilled
- 1¼ teaspoons vanilla extract
- 1 (8 oz.) container low-fat vanilla yogurt
- Orange zest, finely minced, for garnish

## How to Prepare

1. Put water over medium-high heat to boil.

2. Slowly add a couscous, stir once, and remove from heat. Cover and set aside for 12–15 minutes, until the couscous is tender.

3. Add 2 spoons of the sweetener and blend well into the couscous. Cover and hold. Heat juice in a small saucepan over medium heat, stirring constantly until it is reduced to honey consistency (approximately 4–5 minutes).

4. Stir the liqueur back. Set it back. Peel the mango; cut half of the flesh into thin wedges; dice the other half roughly and set aside.

5. Pour the cream in a chilled bowl, whip until it reaches peak. Fold in the vanilla extract and the sweetener remaining. Divide in two and set one bowl aside.

6. Combine remaining half of whipped cream, yogurt, and diced mango in a clean bowl and refrigerate until well chilled.

7. Add mango mixture to couscous before serving. Divide the remaining whipped cream and mango wedges into 6 equal portions, and cover each with a nice dollop.

8. Add liqueur sauce, sprinkle with orange zest, and serve.

## 105.   Fresh Fruit in yogurt with Rum

Serving: 2 Servings

### Ingredients

- ¼ cup each of 2 of the following: blueberries, sliced strawberries, grapes, kiwi, or raspberries
- 2 cups low-fat plain yogurt
- Dark rum (or other favorite liqueur) to taste
- Non-caloric sweetener to taste (optional

## How to Prepare

1. For 2 servings, cut enough necessary or preferred fresh fruit; add 2 cups plain yogurt and stir well.

2. Divide the mixture into 2 individual glass dessert cups and generously sprinkle with dark rum on each serving.

3. If desired, add sweetener; chill over before serving.


## 106.   Fresh Fruit Kebabs and Cinnamon Honey Dip

Serving: 2 Servings

### Ingredients

- Assorted bite-sized chunks of your favorite fresh fruits (enough for 2 8 inch wooden skewers)
- 1 cup low-fat plain yogurt
- 2 tablespoon honey or non-caloric sweetener
- A pinch of ground white pepper
- 6 teaspoon ground cinnamon or to taste

### How to Prepare

1. Prepare fruits and set aside on skewers.

2. Combine yogurt, white pepper and honey, and mix well.

3. Divide the mixture into two individual serving bowls; sprinkle the cinnamon over each serving and swirl gently in.

4. Cover and cool to fridge before serving.


## 107.   Stuffed Dates

Serving: 16 DATES

## Ingredients

- 16 pitted dates
- 16 whole almonds
- 6 tablespoons almond paste

## Instruction

Slice dates open. Take the skin back from the date and stuff 1 almond and 1 tablespoon almond paste for each date. Serve.


## 108.    Sweet Italian rice Pudding

Serving: 6 Servings

## Ingredients

- 24 oz. evaporated skim milk
- ¼ cup long-grain rice
- 3 tablespoons low-calorie baking sweetener
- 1 teaspoon vanilla extract
- Ground cinnamon

## Ingredients

1. Combine the 12 oz. of milk and rice over water in a double boiler. Simmer, sometimes stirring for about 20 minutes.

2. Add remaining sweetener and milk and blend well. Return to a simmer, stirring frequently, until the mixture gains the consistency of a pudding (about 45 minutes).

3. Remove the vanilla extract and blend in the pudding, simmering for a few more minutes. Remove from heat, and generously sprinkle with cinnamon.

4. Cover and refrigerate to room temperature before serving hot.

## 109. Crème de Banana Baked Apples

Serving: 4–6 Serving

**Ingredients**

- 4 medium sweet apples, peeled, cored, and halved
- 6 oz. unsweetened apple juice
- 2 teaspoons ground cinnamon
- 3 tablespoons pure honey
- 1 teaspoon vanilla extract
- 4 tablespoons Crème de Banana liqueur
- 1 cup plain fat-free yogurt
- Non-caloric sweetener to taste

**How to Prepare**

1. Place apples, (cored side up) in a snugly fitting shallow baking dish. Add Apple juice to barely cover the bottom half of apples.

2. Sprinkle with 1 teaspoon of cinnamon, cover and bake in the oven at 350°F (180°C) for 30–40 minutes or until apples are nearly tender.

3. Take out from the oven and empty out any excess liquid, only leaving enough to cover the bottom of the pot. Blend the sugar, vanilla extract and liqueur together, then drizzle over apple tops.

4. Sprinkle the remaining cinnamon spoon over top. Bake for more 10 minutes. Remove from the oven and spread on 4 dessert plates equally. Blend together yogurt and sweetener, and serve side by side.

## 110. Cantaloupe Sorbet

Serving: 4–6 Servings

**Ingredients**

- 1½ cups water
- ½ cup low-calorie baking sweetener
- 2 ripe cantaloupes, peeled, halved, seeded, and chunked
- ¼ cup fresh lemon juice
- ¼ cup egg whites
- Fresh mint sprigs for garnish

**How to Prepare**

1. Combine water and sweetener, and bring to a boil over medium heat. Reduce heat and simmer for 5 minutes, then allow to cool.

2. In a food processor or blender, add cantaloupe and its juices, lemon juice, and cooled syrup. Puree until smooth.

3. Pour mixture into bowl and freeze until almost frozen. Take out from freezer and beat with an electric beater until mixture is again smooth.

4. Beat egg whites until stiff and fold into frozen fruit mixture. Cover container and freeze again until firm (about 2–3 hours).

5. When ready to serve, scoop into dessert cups and garnish with mint sprigs

## 111.    Honeydew Sorbet

Serving: 4–6 Servings

**Ingredients**

- 1½ cups water
- ½ cup low-calorie baking sweetener
- 2 ripe honeydews (about 5 inches in diameter each), peeled, seeded, and chunked
- ¼ cup fresh lemon juice
- ¼ cup egg whites
- Fresh mint sprigs for garnish

**How to Prepare**

1. Combine water and sweetener, and bring to a boil over medium heat. Reduce heat and simmer for 5 minutes, then allow to cool.

2. In a meal processor or blender, include honeydew and its juices, lemon juice, and cooled syrup. Puree until smooth.

3. Pour mixture into bowl and freeze until almost frozen. Withdraw from freezer and beat with an electric beater until mixture is again smooth.

4. Beat egg whites until stiff and fold into frozen fruit mixture.

5. Cover container and freeze again until firm (about 2–3 hours). When ready to serve, scoop into dessert cups and garnish with mint sprigs.


## 112.    Strawberries and Balsamic Syrup

Serving: 4 Serving

**Ingredients**

- 2½ cups fresh strawberries, hulled and halved
- 4 tablespoons Crème de Banana liqueur
- Non-caloric sweetener to taste
- Balsamic syrup

**How to Prepare**

1. In a large bowl, combine strawberries and liqueur, toss well, cover and refrigerate for 20–30 min.

2. Remove strawberries with a slotted spoon when ready to serve and put them on a dessert platter in a single layer.

3. Generously dust with the sweetener, chop with the balsamic syrup and serve.

# 113.    Drunken Peaches

Serving: 4 Servings

## Ingredients

- 4 peaches
- 1½ cups red wine
- 1⅓ cups water
- 3 strips lemon peel (yellow part only)
- 3 tablespoons honey
- 1 cinnamon stick
- Non-caloric sweetener to taste (optional)
- Fat-free whipped cream (optional)

## How to Prepare

1. Peel off peaches skin.

2. Add the wine, sugar, lemon peel, honey, and cinnamon stick in a saucepan and bring to boil.

3. Put the peaches in the saucepan, submerge as much as possible under liquid, and poach gently for 5–10 minutes, until only tender.

4. Remove peaches from saucepan and put them in a bowl; set aside.

5. Boil liquid in a saucepan, continuously stirring until it becomes thick and syrupy.

6. Cut the cinnamon stick and cut the lemon before the liquid darkens.

7. Pour the syrup on top of the peaches and serve when finished. If desired, garnish with sweetener and whipped cream

# 114. Drunken Apricots

Serving: 4 Servings

## Ingredients

- 8 medium apricots
- 1½ cups red wine
- 1⅓ cups water
- 3 strips lemon peel (yellow part only)
- 3 tablespoons honey
- 1 cinnamon stick
- Non-caloric sweetener to taste (optional)
- Fat-free whipped cream (optional)

## How to Prepare

1. Peel the skin from the apricots.

2. Place the wine, sugar, lemon peel, honey, and cinnamon stick in a saucepan and bring to boil.

3. Add the apricots to the sauce, submerge as much as possible under the liquid, and poach gently for 5–10 minutes, until only tender.

4. Remove apricots from saucepan and place them in a bowl; set aside.

5. Boil liquid in a saucepan, continuously stirring until it becomes thick and syrupy.

6. Take out cinnamon stick and lemon peel before liquid becomes dark.

7. Pour syrup, over apricots when cool, and serve. If desired, garnish with sweetener and whipped cream.

# 115. Phyllo Tartlets with Honey Sweetened Cherries

Serving: 8 Tartlets

## Ingredients

- 3 tablespoons instant tapioca
- 5 cups pitted frozen sweet cherries, thawed and drained
- ¾ cup honey, warmed
- 1 tablespoon freshly squeezed lemon juice
- ¾ tablespoon ground cloves
- Pinch of salt
- Butter-flavored cooking spray
- 20 sheets (9x14 inch) phyllo dough, thawed and cut in half

## How to Prepare

1. Process Tapioca in a spice grinder or mini food processor until finely ground.

2. Add the cherries, honey, lemon juice, cloves and salt to a large bowl. Put it aside

3. Preheat oven to 325°F (160°C). Sprinkle lightly with cooking oil on the inside of 8 (3 inches wide) tartlet pans. Unroll phyllo sheets, holding them in a row, on a clean, dry surface.

4. Split the stack cross-sectionally (so you now have 40 sheets).

5. Line sheets with waxed paper and a damp kitchen towel so that they do not dry out while you are working.

6. Place 1 half sheet of phyllo in each saucepan, press it into the bottom, then spray lightly with cooking oil.

7. Continue to add sheets and spray lightly with the cooking oil until 5 layers are in each pan. Trim the phyllo, leaving an overhang of ½ -1 inch.

8. Place the tartlets on a baking sheet. Divide the mixture of cherry between the dishes. Fold the dough over the filling (it will not completely cover).

9. Brush cooking oil gently on the edges of the dough. Cook the tartlets until the filling begins bubbling and the dough is golden brown. Serve when warm.

## 116.    Moroccan Sweet Oranges

Serving: 4 Servings

### Ingredients

- 4 large sweet oranges
- Honey, to drizzle
- Cinnamon, to sprinkle

### How to Prepare

1. Peel the oranges, and slice into rounds crosswise.

2. Arrange orange slices on a dessert plate, sprinkle honey and cinnamon over the tops and serve.

## 117.    Pumpkin Pudding

Serving: 4 Servings

### Ingredients

- 1¾ cups skim milk
- 1 (1 oz.) package no sugar instant vanilla pudding mix
- ½ cup canned pumpkin
- ½ teaspoon pumpkin spice

### How to Prepare

1. In a chilled cup, add cold milk and pudding mixture, and stir until smooth.

2. Add in the pumpkin and spice, and cool before serving to chill.

## 118.  Honey Nests

Serving: 4 Servings

**Ingredients**

- ½ pound angel hair pasta
- 8 tablespoons trans-fat–free canola/olive oil spread, melted
- 1½ cups shelled pistachio nuts, chopped, divided
- ¼ cup low-calorie baking sweetener
- ⅓ cup honey
- ⅝ cup water
- 2 teaspoons freshly squeezed lemon juice
- Low-fat plain Greek yogurt for garnish

**How to Prepare**

1. Preheat the oven to 350°F (180°C).

2. Cook pasta as instructed by package and drain thoroughly. Transfer the pasta into a bowl and add the spread of melted canola/olive oil.

3. Toss the pasta to coat and let it cool. Divide the pasta into eight equal servings.

4. Use 4 small oven-safe bowls, gently press 1 serving of pasta down into each of the 4 bowls and top with half of the nuts.

5. Cover each with a portion of pasta left over and put bowls on a baking sheet. Bake for 45 minutes, or till golden brown and crispy on top of the pasta.

6. While cooking the pasta, mix sweetener, honey and water in a small saucepan and bring to a boil at low heat, continuously stirring until sweetener is dissolved.

7. Let it boil for another 10 minutes, add lemon juice and cook for another 5 minutes.

8. When pasta is well browned (not burned), remove angel hair nests from the oven and carefully pass them to serve dishes.

9. Drizzle honey lemon over nest tops and sprinkle with remaining nuts. Allow to cool with a dollop of yogurt before serving.

## 119.  Strawberry Rhubarb Quinoa Pudding

Serving: 6 Servings

### Ingredients

- 3 cups water, divided
- 1½ cups chopped rhubarb, fresh or frozen
- 1 cup chopped strawberries, fresh or frozen, + more for garnish
- ½ cup quinoa
- ½ teaspoon ground cinnamon
- Dash of salt
- ¼ cup + 1½ teaspoons low-calorie baking sweetener
- ½ teaspoon freshly grated lemon zest
- 1 tablespoon cornstarch
- 1 cup plain non-fat yogurt
- 1 teaspoon pure vanilla extract

### How to Prepare

1. Combine 2¾ cups tea, rhubarb, strawberries, quinoa, cinnamon and salt into a saucepan.

2. Bring to a boil, and lower to a simmer liquid.

3. Cover and cook for about 25 minutes, or until the quinoa is tender. Stir in lemon zest and ¼ cup sweetener.

4. Combine the remaining ¼ cup water with cornstarch and whisk until smooth in a small bowl, then add to the quinoa mixture and let simmer, stirring constantly for 1 minute.

5. Remove from heat, divide between 6 serving bowls and wait for 1 hour to cool.

6. Alternatively, in a small bowl, mix the yogurt, vanilla extract, and remaining 1½ teaspoon sweetener.

7. Finish each serving with a generous dollop of yogurt blend and fresh sliced strawberries.

## 120.    Drunken Strawberries

Serving: 4 Servings

**Ingredients**

- 1 pound hulled fresh strawberries, sliced
- 1½ packets of a non-caloric sweetener
- 1 tablespoon Grand Marnier liqueur
- 1 teaspoon freshly squeezed lemon juice
- 1 cup low-fat plain Greek yogurt

**How to Prepare**

1. In a dish, mix strawberries, sweetener, liqueur and lemon juice.

2. Let stand and marinate, approximately 10–15 minutes, before strawberries release their juices.

3. Divide the mixture into four bowls for dessert, add ¼ cup yogurt to each bowl and serve.

# 121.   Deliciously Sweetened Yogurt

Serving: 2 Servings

## Ingredients

- 2 ripe apricots, halved, pitted, and cut to ½ inch wedges
- 1 cup sweet cherries, halved and pitted
- 3 teaspoons fresh mint, finely chopped
- 6 packets non-caloric sweetener, divided
- 2 cups low-fat plain Greek yogurt
- 2 teaspoons pure vanilla extract
- 2 tablespoons shelled, chopped, and toasted pistachios

## How to Prepare

1. Mix apricots, tart cherries, basil, and 1½ sweetener packets together.

2. Let stand for 10 to 15 minutes until some of their juices are released by the fruits. In the meantime, mix cereal, vanilla extract and remaining sweetener. Mix until smooth and blended

3. . Divide the yogurt mixture into 2 bowls and finish with a combination of fruit and nuts. Serve right away.


# 122.   Easy Peach Cobbler

Serving: 15 Servings

## Ingredients

- ½ cup + 1½ teaspoons low-calorie baking sweetener
- 2 tablespoons cornstarch
- 1 (29 oz.) can sliced peaches, drained, liquid reserved
- ½ tablespoon ground cinnamon
- 2 tablespoon trans-fat–free canola/olive oil spread
- 1 cup self-rising flour

- 1 tablespoon trans-fat–free shortening
- ½ cup almond milk

**How to Prepare**

1. Preheat oven to 400°F (200°C) .

2. Combine ½ cup sweetener and cornstarch in a saucepan, stirring gradually in reserved peach juice and bringing to a boil for 1 minute, constantly stirring.

3. Add peaches, pour in a 9x13 inch baking dish, sprinkle with cinnamon, spread canola/olive oil line, and set aside.

4. Mix the flour with the remaining sweetener, cut with shortening, then add the milk and stir until all the ingredients are well blended.

5. Spoon the dough on the fruit and bake for 25-30 minutes. Serve hot.

## 123.　Lemon Cakes

Serving: 8 Servings

**Ingredients**

- 2 tablespoon trans-fat–free canola/olive oil spread + more, softened, to coat ramekins
- ⅓ cup all-purpose flour, spooned and leveled
- ½ teaspoon baking powder
- ¼ teaspoon salt
- 3 large eggs, separated
- ¼ cup + ⅛ cup low-calorie baking sweetener
- 1 teaspoon finely grated lemon zest
- ⅓ cup freshly squeezed lemon juice
- 1¼ cups almond milk

- Confectioners' sugar for dusting, scant amount

**How to Prepare**

1. Preheat oven to 325°F (160°C).

2. Brush 8 (6 oz.) ramekins with softened canola/olive oil spread applied to the sides and bottoms.

3. Place the ramekins in a shallow casserole dish for baking.

4. Put together flour, baking powder and salt in a dish. Whisk together egg yolks with ¼ cup sweetener in a separate larger bowl, until the mixture is light and smooth.

5. Whisk the canola/olive oil, lemon zest, lemon juice, milk and flour mixture in 2 tablespoons. Cover the mixture and cool for 3 hours.

6. Beat the egg whites (using an electric mixer) in another large bowl with ⅛ cup sweetener until it forms peaks, about 5 minutes, and fold into chilled batter. Divide batter among ramekins with a ladle, wiping away any excess dripped from the edges.

7. Add sufficient water to the casserole dish so it comes halfway up the ramekin sides.

8. Place the casserole dish with the ramekins in the oven and bake for about 30 minutes until the cakes puff and are somewhat golden on top.

9. Dust with the confectioner's sugar and serve hot.


## 124.    Vanilla-Rhubarb Compote

Serving: 4 Servings

**Ingredients**

- 4 cups diced rhubarb

- ¼ cup low-calorie baking sweetener
- ¼ teaspoon ground cinnamon
- ½ teaspoon pure vanilla extract
- 4 (store-bought) crêpes
- Vanilla yogurt or fat-free ice cream for serving

## How to Prepare

1. Combine the rhubarb, sweetener, and cinnamon in a saucepan.

2. Bring to a simmer over medium-high heat, then reduce heat to low simmer and cook until the rhubarb starts breaking down, around 5 minutes.

3. Remove from heat and add vanilla extract at low-medium heat, combine orange juice and sweetener in a saucepan.

4. Cook, stirring constantly, for about 3 minutes, before sweetener dissolves. Add the yogurt and vanilla extract, then swirl to blend. Transfer into a large spouted container and fill 10 ice-pop molds (3 oz.).

5. Add popsicle sticks and freeze for close to 6 hours, or as long as 1 week, until the pops are firm.

6. Briefly run molds under hot water to detach pops and extract it from molds.

## 125.  Strawberry-Walnut Trifle

Serving: 15 Servings

## Ingredients

- 1 small, no-sugar-added angel food cake
- 3 oz. sugar-free strawberry gelatin
- 10 oz. frozen, unsweetened strawberries, thawed and halved (reserve 1 cup for garnish)
- 2 bananas, sliced

- 1 (1½ oz.) package sugar-free instant vanilla pudding mix
- 3 cups almond milk
- Fat-free whipped cream
- Chopped walnut pieces, to sprinkle

**How to Prepare**

1. Tear cake into bite size pieces and place in a glass trifle bowl.

2. Dissolve the gelatin in 1 cup boiling water and apply to the strawberries. Using a spoon, spread the strawberries uniformly over pieces of cake.

3. Put banana slices to the top of the strawberries and cool down as pudding is being prepared. Combine the pudding mixture with the almond milk and whisk until it starts to set for about 2 minutes.

4. Refrigerate pudding to set more firmly for an additional 5 minutes before adding it to the trifle cup, spooning evenly over bananas and strawberries.

5. Trifle bowl mixture should be refrigerated at least 2 hours before serving.

6. Finish with reserved strawberries, a dollop of whipped cream and a sprinkle of chopped walnuts each serving.

## 126.    Homestyle apple pie

Serving: 8 Servings

**Ingredients**

**For Crust**

- 1 cup pastry flour
- 6 tablespoons canola oil
- 3 tablespoons water

- All-purpose flour

## For Filling

- 6 sweet apples, cored, peeled, and sliced (Red or Yellow Delicious, Gala, or Macintosh)
- ⅔ cup low-calorie baking sweetener
- ⅛ teaspoon salt
- ¾ teaspoon cinnamon
- ¾ teaspoon nutmeg
- 1½ tablespoons trans-fat–free canola oil/olive oil spread
- Fat-free whipped cream (optional)

## How to Prepare

### Crust

1. Prepare dough with the canola oil and water by mixing pastry flour. Mix well and turn it into a ball.

2. Use a small quantity of all-purpose flour to cover the work surface, put the dough on the surface and sprinkle a small quantity of all-purpose flour on the dough.

3. Roll the dough out into a wide enough flat circle to cover the inside and sides of a 9 inch pie pan.

### Filling

1. Place sliced apples in a bowl, add sweetener, salt, cinnamon and nutmeg and stir to coat dried ingredients on apple slices. Move apple to dough lined pie pan.

2. Spread the apples evenly out. Place the canola/olive oil dots scattered over the apple top and place the pie in the oven.

3. Bake for 15 minutes, at 450°F.

4. Reduce the oven to 350°F (180°C) and bake another 45 minutes.

5. Remove from the oven and gently cool before cutting. When needed, serve warm with fat-free whipped cream.

## 127. Espresso Granita

Serving: 6 servings

**Ingredients**

- ½ cup water
- ½ cup sugar
- 2 cups espresso
- ½ teaspoon real vanilla
- Whipped cream for topping (optional)

**How to Prepare**

1. Place water and sugar in a small casserole and heat over medium heat until it boils, about ten minutes, stirring occasionally. Do not be tempted by heating on high to intensify this, as the sugar will burn. Boil the sugar mixture without stirring for 5 minutes, then remove it from heat. Replace once and allow to completely cool.

2. In a lightweight casserole dish or baking pan (not aluminum), add the espresso, sugar syrup and vanilla. Put in the fridge.

3. Extract and swirl the crystals around the edges with a fork in the center after 30 minutes. Place in freezer again. Remove pan and mix crystals with a fork every 30 minutes. Make use of the side of a spoon to shave the bigger chunks if you miss and wait too long.

4. When the granita is done completely frozen (4–6 hours). You can keep it in a refrigerator for a day or two, covered, but occasionally stir it to keep it from freezing up into a hard slab. When they are ready to serve, spoon granita into wine or champagne glasses. When needed, top off with whipped cream.

# 128. Honey Sweetened Broiled-Feta

Serving: 4 servings

## Ingredients

- 12 oz. feta cheese cut into 3 × ½ inch sticks
- 1 tablespoon extra virgin olive oil
- ¼ cup honey
- ½ teaspoon aniseed

## How to Prepare

1. Fill broiler with preheat. Divide cheese sticks between four ceramic ramekins that are broiler-proof. Brush oil to the cheese.

2. Place ramekins under the broiler, approximately 6 inches from source heat.

3. Broil about 2–4 minutes till the cheese is golden brown and bubbly.

4. Watch it closely because this is going to happen quickly, and you don't want the cheese to burn. Take ramekins off and put to one side.

5. Mix honey and aniseed in a small saucepan and heat until hot over medium heat or combine for 90 seconds at 50 percent power in a glass measuring cup and heat in the microwave.

6. Finish each serving of the honey mixture with equal portions of cheese. Serve straightaway.


# 129. Wine-Stewed Figs with Yogurt Cream

Serving: 4 servings

## Ingredients

- ½ cup brown sugar
- 1 bottle of red table wine (or 4 cups cranberry juice)
- Juice and zest from 1 organic lemon
- 2 cinnamon sticks
- 3 cloves
- 2 pounds fresh figs
- 2 cups plain low-fat or non fat yogurt
- 1 teaspoon vanilla
- 1 tablespoon honey
- Ground cinnamon for garnish

## How to Prepare

1. Mix brown sugar, wine (or cranberry juice), lemon juice and zest, cinnamon sticks, and cloves into a large stainless steel or non-stick saucepan.

2. Heat up over medium-high heat until the liquid boils. Reduce heat to medium and cook, constantly stirring, until the mixture begins to thicken slightly, and the sugar is completely dissolved.

3. Lower to low-medium heat, and add figs to the mixture of wine, stirring gently to cover figs. Simmer 5 minutes in wine mixture, continually stirring to keep the figs going and coated.

4. Take figs off in a glass or ceramic bowl.

5. Continue to cook the wine until it's shrunk by about half and appears like a thin syrup. Take out the sticks and cloves of cinnamon, and discard.

6. Ladle the syrup from the wine over the figs. Chill a total of 1 hour in the refrigerator.

7. Place them in 4 individual dessert dishes or bowls when you are ready to serve the figs. Drizzle the figs over any remaining syrup.

8. Place the yoghurt in a medium bowl. Spray with cinnamon and honey.

9. Stir and mix gently. Finish each fig platter with some yogurt cream. Sprinkle and serve each with the ground cinnamon.

## 130.   Orange Banana Muffins

Serving: 12 servings

**Ingredients**

- 3 cups rolled oats
- ½ cup almonds
- 1 tablespoon baking powder
- 1 egg
- 1 very ripe banana, mashed
- 1 cup mandarin orange slices, drained and mashed with a fork
- 1 cup unsweetened applesauce
- ½ cup canned pumpkin puree (not pumpkin pie mixture)
- ½ cup brown sugar
- 1 tablespoon vanilla
- ½ cup non-fat plain yogurt

**How to Prepare**

1. Preheat oven to 375°F (190°C).

2. Place the oats and almonds in a blender and grind into a flour.

3. Pour into a large bowl to blend. Stir in baking powder and mix. Beat the egg using a fork in a different dish. In addition, add bananas, grapes, applesauce, pumpkin and sugar. Mix well with a fork, until fully combined.

4. Stir the vanilla into the yogurt into 2 cups of water.

5. Add one-third of oat mixture to the banana mixture. Stir till combined. Add half the yogurt and whisk until the yogurt is combined. Repeat the remaining yogurt and the remaining oat mixture with another third of the oat mixture.

6. Spray 12 nonstick-cooking spray muffin cups or use muffin liners. Fill batter with muffin cups. Bake for 20 minutes, or until set in the middle. Remove from the oven, cool and remove from muffin tin for 15 minutes.

7. Completely cool before serving.

## 131.  Lemon Almond Cake

Serving: 4 to 5 servings

**Ingredients**

- 1½ cups blanched almonds
- ¼ cup honey
- 4 large eggs
- Zest from 2 organic lemons
- ¼ teaspoon nutmeg

**How to Prepare**

1. Preheat oven to 375°F (190°C). Spray nonstick cooking spray on a 9 inch springform tin.

2. In a food processor or blender, put the almonds and grind to a fine meal.

3. Split the eggs and place yolks in a large mixing bowl, and the whites in a separate, clean mixing bowl. Then apply the sugar, zest, then nutmeg to the yolks. Beat on medium just below the surface of the yolk to increase the thickness of the mixture, around 3 minutes.

4. Completely clean the beaters and beat the egg whites until soft peaks are formed.

5. Stir almonds into the yolk mixture, then fold in the egg whites. Scoop the batter gently into the springform tin.

6. Bake for 30–40 minutes until a toothpick inserted in the cake's center comes out clean.

7. Cool down for 5 minutes. Detached the edges of the cake from the sides of the pan using a sharp knife. Cool for another 25 minutes, then cut sides. Serve with ice cream, at room temperature.

## 132. Critics Compote

Serving: 6 servings

### Ingredients

- 2 medium tangerines
- 2 medium size oranges
- 1 medium size red grapefruit
- 1 medium size of lemon at room temperature
- 1 medium size lime at room temperature
- 1-2 teaspoon sugar (optional)
- Fresh coconut slivers or cut off almonds for garnish (non-compulsory)

### How to Prepare

1. Peel the bananas, tangerines and grapefruit. Segment and remove the white pith trim. (You don't have to cut everything off because pith is loaded with the phytochemicals and fiber. However, too much pith adds a bitter taste.)

2. Halve or quarter any segments bigger than bite-sized segments.

3. With a sharp knife, cut out any seeds. In a large bowl, combine the segments.

4. Quarter the lemon and lime, then squeeze over the citrus pieces. And halve and use a juicer to remove the juice, then drizzle over the segments of the citrus.

5. Sprinkle with sugar if necessary and blend gently. Chill for a total of 1 hour, and drink cold.

6. Serve in wine glasses. Garnish with coconut slivers or chopped almond sprinkling, if desired.


## 133.  Baked Apples and Pears

Serving: 8 Servings

### Ingredients

- ½ cup brown sugar
- ¼ cup chopped walnuts, almonds, or a combination
- ¼ cup raisins or dried currants
- 4 medium-large apples
- 4 medium pears, still firm
- 1-2 tablespoons freshly squeezed lemon juice
- 2 cups red wine, apple cider, or apple juice
- ½ teaspoon ground cinnamon
- A quarter teaspoon grounded nutmeg
- Rind from 1 small well-wash, naturally grown orange or lemon, cut in strips

### How to Prepare

1. Preheat oven to 300°F (150°C).

2. Blend ¼ cup brown sugar, nuts, and raisins in a small bowl. Put aside.

3. Core the apples from the top, leaving an apple about ½ inch at the root. The pears don't center but slice off the very bottoms so that they stand up straight. Keep the roots flawless.

4. Brush any peel off or cut fruit surfaces with lemon juice, then put the fruits in a 1-1½ quarter baking pot or saucepan. Fill the apples with the mixture of the nut.

5. Combine the wine, vinegar or juice in a saucepan with the cinnamon, nutmeg, the remaining brown sugar, and the rind of citrus. Heat to simmer, then sprinkle carefully over the berries.

6. Close the pan with a lid or foil made of aluminum, then bake for 30 to 45 minutes until the fruit is soft when pierced with a fork. Baste regularly when baking with the wine sauce.

7. Serve each piece of fruit with the wine sauce spooned over the top, in a shallow bowl or small dish. They also look beautifully served in wine glasses or stemmed glass sundae.

## 134.  Macedonian Salad (A "Spirited" Fruit Salad)

Serving: 6 servings

### Ingredients

- A lemon brought to room temperature
- A cup cubed peaches or nectarines
- A cup strawberries, halved, or other berries
- 1 cup seedless grapes (green, red, or a combination)
- 1 cup melon cubes or balls (cantaloupe, honeydew, or watermelon)
- ¼ cup sugar (optional, but it brings out the juice)
- ½ cup red wine (try a Zinfandel for a rich, peppery effect, a Pinot Noir for a lighter, flowery taste) or

- 2 tablespoon liqueur (Grand Marnier, kirsch, or amaretto are all good choices) or ½ cup orange juice

**How to Prepare**

1. Gently roll the lemon on the counter and cut it into quarters. Put it aside.

2. In a large bowl, combine the remaining fruit gently and squeeze each quarter of the lemon over the fruit immediately, stirring gently to keep the fruit from breaking or mashing.

3. Sprinkle with the sugar, then substitute the champagne, liqueur, or orange juice. Gently set fire to the liqueur if desired.

4. Allow 10 to 15 minutes (no more than 1 hour) to sit at room temperature, then serve.

# CONCLUSION

The Mediterranean diet meal plan is very easy to follow since the food selection includes full flavor oils, whole breads and cereals, fruits, vegetables, nuts, seeds, beans and a host of hunger-blasting foods. But perhaps the best advantage of adopting a Mediterranean diet meal plan is how easy it is to lose pounds of unhealthy fat in the belly.

Wherever you hold your extra pounds of fat, your overall health appearance will make a big difference. Too much belly fat induces crowding of your internal organs and this causes a chain reaction of poor health effects from increased levels of LDL (bad) cholesterol to high blood pressure, diabetes, and heart disease.

The Mediterranean diet mainly consists of organic, healthy plant foods, such as whole grains, vegetables, fruits, nuts, legumes, olives, fish and seafood. We pair this with small quantities of red meat and dairy products.

The Mediterranean diet is more balanced due to the less processed foods. It deprives it of nutrients by processing food, and even cooking it. But most foods are eaten raw or lightly cooked in a typical Mediterranean diet, too. Normally trimmed with excess fat while serving red meat. The overall diet provides the body with ample food, healthy fats, vitamins, minerals, calcium, and essential fatty acids needed to maintain health and prevent chronic diseases such as heart disease and cancer.

When you take a tape measure and loop it around your belly at the point just above your hip bones, and weigh more than 40 inches if you're a man or more than 35 inches if you're a woman, that means you need a healthy diet change and the solution may be following a Mediterranean diet meal plan.

Following the measures and meal plan outlined in this book is a healthy way to lose both belly fat and weight from other body areas. The diet is naturally high in fiber, vitamins, nutrients, and minerals, thereby strengthening the heart when you lose weight. Isn't that a better side effect than taking a drug for weight loss?

Is your stomach too big? Are you concerned you've let your weight go too far and now feel stressed and anxious about what you're going to do in the future to get rid of this stomach fat?

I know how scary this can be and what I don't want you to do is hop on the band wagon of some stupid fad diet that promises a super-fast weight loss, but it ends up leaving you feeling tired, moody and completely starving.

Stop chasing fast solutions, and get the answer.

Whether you are searching for a healthy way to live and eat, or you are looking for a diet that will help you lose weight, the Mediterranean Diet is a good choice. With this diet you will not drop 20 pounds in a month, but it will help you get to and sustain a very healthy weight. This is not just a diet you begin and end but also a way to change the way you eat for the rest of your life every single day.

It's nice to find a diet that doesn't cut stuff you should enjoy to the max. You can still have red meat, just not that often and with this diet you are even allowed to drink wine. Most diets don't allow alcohol and will take out a lot of the things you need. With the Mediterranean Diet, you can have confidence in knowing you're eating healthily in a hearth way that fully supports your body.